RAY KYBARTAS

with Kenneth Ross

Introduction by Madonna

Art Direction and Design: Ross Patrick

Photography: Jeff Higginbotham

Simon & Schuster

FITNESS
IS RELIGION

KEEP THE
FAITH

SIMON & SCHUSTER
Rockefeller Center
1230 Avenue of the Americas, New York, NY 10020

Art direction and design by Ross Patrick
Photographs copyright © 1997 by Jeff Higginbotham

Manufactured in the United States of America

1 3 5 7 9 10 8 6 4 2

Library of Congress Cataloging-in-Publication Data
Kybartas, Ray.
Fitness is religion—keep the faith / Ray Kybartas with Kenneth
Ross; photography, Jeff Higginbotham.
p. cm.
1. Physical fitness. 2. Nutrition. 3. Physical fitness—Psychological aspects.
I. Ross, Kenneth, date. II. Title.
GV481.K93 1997
613.7—dc21   97-31490   CIP

ISBN 0-684-84211-4

In view of the complex, individual, and specific nature of health and
fitness problems, this book, and the ideas, programs, procedures, and suggestions
in it, are not intended to replace the advice of trained medical professionals.
All matters regarding one's health require medical supervision. A physician
should be consulted prior to adopting any program described in the book if the
reader has any condition that may require diagnosis or medical attention.
The authors and publisher disclaim any liability arising
directly or indirectly from the use of this book.

The chapter entitled Practical Matters is taken in large part from
the booklet *Better Health with Balance*, published by Bio-Foods, Inc.,
makers of the Balance nutrition bar and other nutritional products.

Acknowledgments

My first thanks are to Madonna and all my clients for their constant encouragement and enduring loyalty. I could not have written this book without the benefit of their inspiration and ongoing commitment to health and fitness.

Many people have made significant contributions to this book. I would like to thank Michael Sanchez for his expert help in preparing the chapter on nutrition, and for his many other helpful suggestions. Michael, who is a Feldenkrais practitioner, also provided the material on the Feldenkrais method. The menus in this book are courtesy of Bio Foods Corporation, maker of Balance bars and other nutritional products. I would like to thank Denise Kaufman and John Casey for their help in preparing the section on yoga, and Karyn Klein for her assistance in preparing the section on the Pilates method.

I also want to thank the models, amateur and professional, who agreed to be photographed for this book: Claudia Compos, Eloise DeJoria, Woody Gair, John Montanaro, Mike Newman, Ingo Radamacher, and David Rosen. My thanks also to Gold's Gym for the use of their facility, and the Asics, Adidas, Cannondale, and Oakley companies for the use of their products.

To Debbie, Jessie, and Shayne

Contents

INTRODUCTION

by Madonna

The first time I met Ray I was in Tennessee visiting my future husband who is now my ex-husband on the set of his movie *At Close Range*. I think I was getting on Sean's nerves (there's not a lot to do on the set of a movie even if you're in it), and he suggested I go for a run with the trainer he had hired to make him look like a hunk in the film. Ray showed up at my hotel as I was lacing my sneakers.

I don't know how we ended up on the dirt road that went on for miles. We could have driven there in his truck. We could have walked. Maybe we flew. The thing is, as soon as Ray showed up, I forgot that I was about to do something difficult. After all it was the middle of summer and 90 degrees in the shade.

First of all he was so damn cheerful. Second of all he was tan and fit and absolutely radiated good health. And last but certainly not least he was so innocent. About everything. Women, money, the entertainment business. I could go on and on. He didn't even swear. In the beginning I used to try and bribe him with money to say a teeny tiny four letter word. But he would just blush. He was so adorable. I couldn't believe he was from L.A.

We talked about women—he needed to have more confidence. We talked about money—I told him to ask for more. We talked about the entertainment business—no free rides, never trust anyone, watch your back, etc., etc. I was feeling very experienced and jaded.

Then he picked up the pace. I had to work hard to keep up with him, and I was definitely sucking air, but he made me laugh so hard

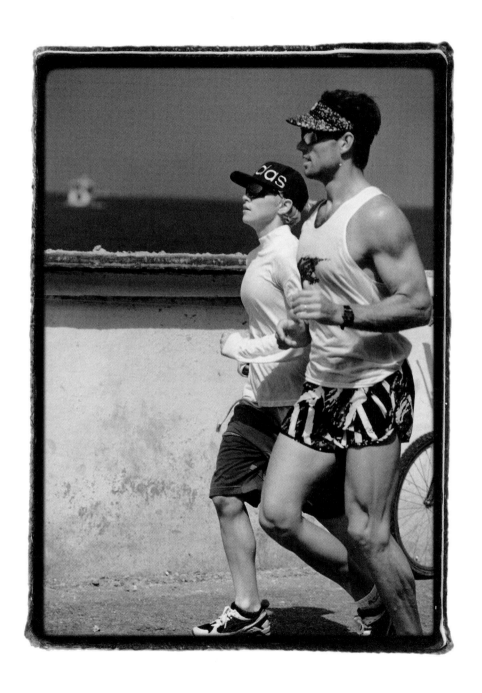

with his silly anecdotes that I didn't realize I was suffering. We finished the run, and I felt invigorated. That's when I first realized that it was possible to exercise and enjoy yourself.

Ray and I worked out a few more times, and I went back on the road to finish a tour. Eventually I returned home to L.A. and decided I wanted to get a trainer full time. I tried several, but none of them made the impact that Ray had. None of them made me laugh. None of them motivated me the way Ray did. I picked up the phone, dialed his number, and I've been training with him ever since.

Some days we run forever. Some days we ride bikes. Some days we swim and run stairs. Some days we do weight training. Some days we have a pancake breakfast, and lately we've been doing lots of yoga. He makes working out fun and encourages me to rest when I'm burned out. The important thing is variety and adapting it to my lifestyle.

There are no rules. All you need is dedication. That's where the whole church thing came into our fitness vocabulary. I don't know who started it, me or Ray, but we were in Indiana filming *A League of Their Own*. Once again it was the middle of summer, and I had to look like I played baseball for a living.

We were training like maniacs. Filming started at 8 A.M. so we had to get up at 5 to get a workout in. It would still be dark out. The phone would ring, and I'd hear Ray's voice cackling like a witch at the other end of the line, "Evilsky, are you ready for church?" You have to imagine Boris Karloff after too many cups of coffee to get the full effect.

Sometimes it was so dark we'd run into telephone poles or trip on fresh roadkill. We'd make ourselves feel better by exclaiming that nobody else had "the religion."

There were lots of other movie sets and concert tours that we've been together on, and I give Ray a lot of credit for keeping my spirits up and injecting levity into working situations that inevitably became grueling experiences. I will always be indebted to him for keeping me in good shape and teaching me about proper nutrition, but more important, for keeping my head in a good place. Whether we're doing windsprints uphill or sun salutes in my living room, the goal has been much more about peace of mind than having a perfect body.

Physical beauty is ephemeral, but the self-confidence and emotional strength one builds from achieving difficult things and accomplishing goals is the most beautiful thing of all.

The important thing is to have fun while you're doing it. To enjoy the journey. That's what life's all about.

That's what this book is all about.

♡ Madonna

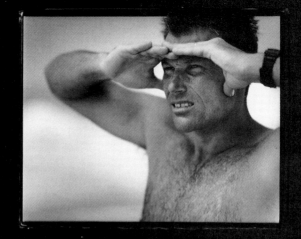

LEAP OF FAITH

I am a first-generation American, the son of Lithuanian immigrants. And like my parents, my life has been inalterably shaped by a journey—not a geographical one, but a pilgrimage of personal growth and achievement. My own pilgrimage has transformed me from a shy and overweight underachiever, to the heights of my profession. Yet as I look back, I can hardly believe it has happened. When I was young, no one—least of all me—thought I would succeed at anything. I grew up a chubby, out of shape kid in Santa Monica, California. My older brother, Ed, was the athlete in the family. Ed had a legendary career at Santa Monica High School playing football. He went on to be a college All American. When I entered high school, the coaches assumed that I carried the same genetic heritage as my brother, and recruited me to follow in his footsteps. I couldn't do it. My family, friends, and coaches didn't understand what was wrong with me. They all labeled me an underachiever.

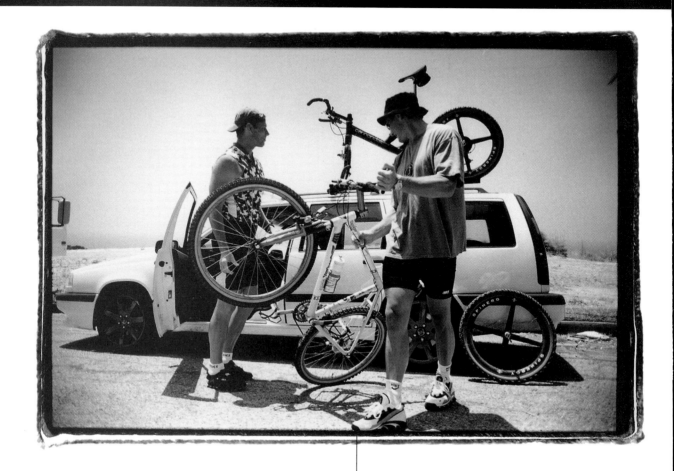

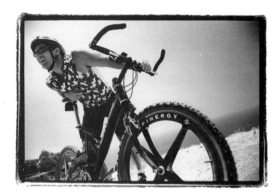

up at dawn

An early morning ride is like an act of
devotion. It centers the mind for the
day to come.

W H A T
TIME IS CHURCH?

When Madonna calls me to confirm our workout schedule she often asks the question, "What time's church?" For her, fitness is a religion, a way of life rooted in the deeply held conviction that physical, psychological, and spiritual health are inextricably related.

"Beauty is superficial and fleeting, but health is profound and lasting."

Madonna shares my belief that the pursuit of fitness is the pursuit of wholeness, a religious regimen that can empower each of us to cope with the overwhelming pressures of our day-to-day existence. "Ray," Madonna said to me once, "if I didn't work out with you, I just wouldn't *feel* right!" The religious fervor that she invests in her fitness program helps her to ward off anger, anxiety, and fatigue and enables her to cope with a grueling schedule.

For Madonna and my other clients, the cosmetic benefits of a fitness program are not the primary reason they exercise. In fact, vanity is a secondary motive. They all want to look good, but it is *health* they seek. Beauty is superficial and fleeting, but health is profound and lasting.

Vanity is never satisfied when it is the primary focus of any fitness program. Genuine beauty is the result of a larger commitment.

"We must be transformed from the inside out."

Fitness is a lifelong pilgrimage. And like religious pilgrims, all who seek health must commit themselves to the journey. Those who do will find lasting results. Here is the irony: To achieve physical beauty you must look beyond it. If we keep our eyes focused on a particular short-term goal we may achieve it, but the victory will be temporary. We must be transformed from the inside out.

Mike Newman, a forty-year-old world-class athlete (and actor on *Baywatch*), like Madonna, has made a long-term commitment. And like her, when he talks about fitness, the religious metaphors slip easily into his speech. We were jogging together one day on the beach, when he said, "You know, Ray, I think athletes fall into two groups: the believers and the nonbelievers. The nonbelievers just want to win the race, but they never seem to enjoy training for it. And you know what? Nonbelievers seldom last. The glory of winning is so short-lived. The people with staying power—the believers—have a passion for the process. They enjoy winning, but they cherish the athletic lifestyle even more."

"In fitness, as in religion, you must make the leap of faith."

Of course, he is right. The "unbelievers" are like people who go to a church—or temple or mosque—but only on religious holidays. Then they wonder why their spiritual lives never develop! All religious traditions recognize that there is no growth without commitment, and no commitment without belief. In fitness, as in religion, you must make the leap of faith.

I know people who have kept the faith all of their lives. Early in my career I managed the original Gold's Gym in Santa Monica, California. There was a man in his seventies who worked out there at the time. He was something of a legend at Gold's. He had a physique that was the envy of most twenty-year-olds. That old man never missed a workout. He was completely dedicated to a healthy lifestyle and had little patience for those who thought fitness could be achieved overnight. Like an old biblical prophet who had achieved wisdom the hard way, he could be a little cranky.

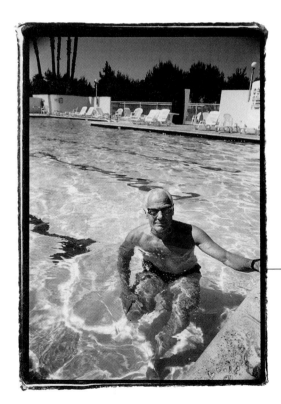

keeping the faith

Sixty-seven-year-old Woody Gair swims ninety minutes four times a week, and competes regularly at the master's level. Woody is still young in mind, body, and spirit.

YOU MUST KEEP THE FAITH

One morning a young man in his twenties came in and enrolled at the gym. Looking around, he saw the older man across the room, working out. His face and physique didn't seem to go together. His gray head was that of a well-kept septuagenarian, but his body seemed grafted on—impossibly young looking. In his sweatpants and tank shirt, his exposed arms and shoulders revealed full, deeply defined muscles covered with smooth, tight skin. There wasn't an ounce of fat on him. Awestruck, the young man walked over to him and said, "You look great, how long have you been working out?" The old man gave him a fierce look and replied, "All my damned life—you're looking at a *lifetime* of working out!"

"There are no shortcuts."

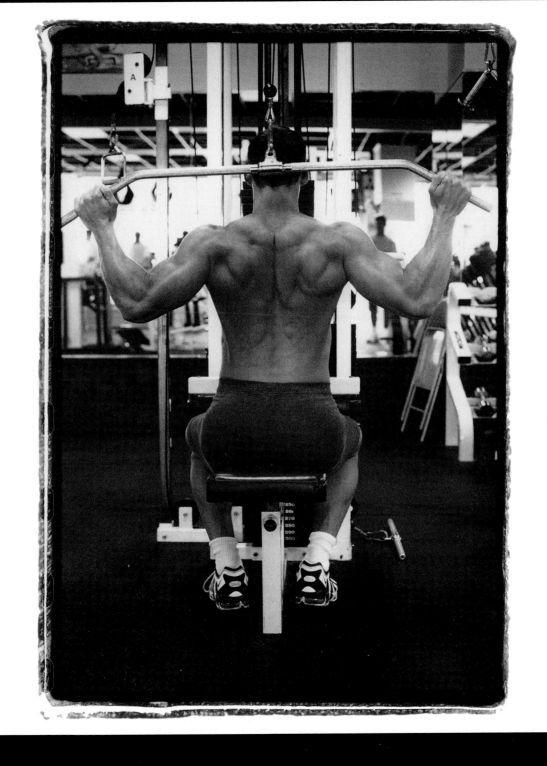

The old guy knew what most people were looking for—a quick fix, a magic formula, or some well-kept secret, and it irritated him greatly. He knew what believers everywhere know: There are no shortcuts. Here, he thought, was one more fool hoping to achieve in six months what was, in fact, a life's work.

Long-term goals are not popular with most of us. In a society as fast paced and transient as ours, the idea of anything constituting a life's work is rare. We want immediate results, a quick turnaround, a prompt return on our investment. Corporations are obsessed with quarterly reports, investors with short-term gains, entrepreneurs with a fast buck. We all want instant success. Is it any wonder that we expect the same from our bodies?

Fad diets, liposuction, drug-assisted weight loss, crash exercise programs—all these and more—hold out the promise of instant results. In Southern California where I live, I have seen posters for a weight-loss clinic stapled to telephone poles near freeway off-ramps, advertising: LOSE THIRTY POUNDS IN THIRTY DAYS! The fact that it might take thirty weeks (or even thirty months) to lose that much weight safely was of little concern to that clinic.

"Our neglected bodies often serve only as a repository for stress, depression, and illness."

Instant weight loss is not commensurate with health. With the *long-term* pursuit of fitness, however, weight loss, or more precisely *fat* loss, takes care of itself—automatically. Again, to achieve it you must not pursue it! The object is not to lose weight but to become fit.

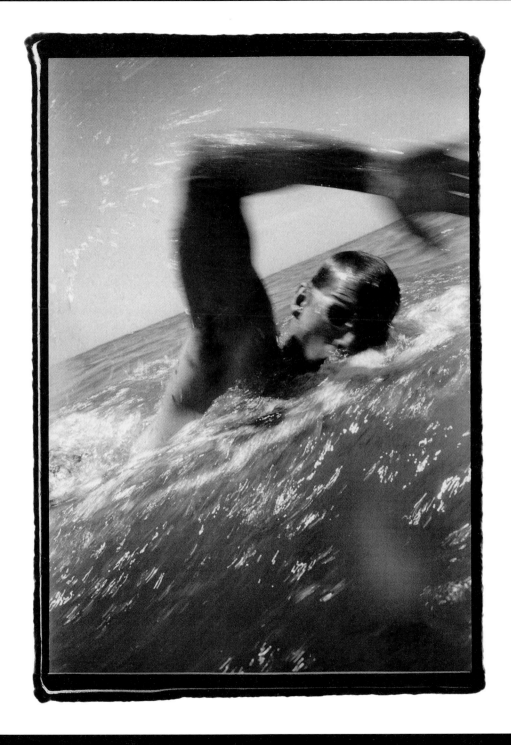

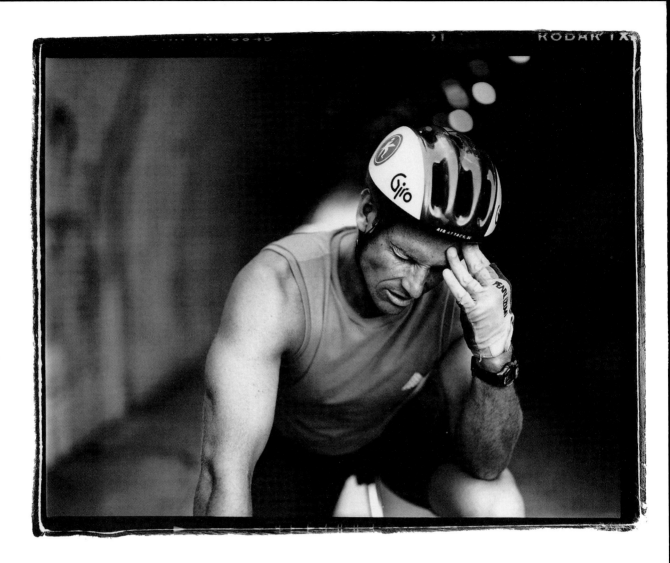

"We seldom make the connections between our physical health and our spiritual well-being."

WE HAVE DISASSOCIATED HEALTH FROM BEAUTY

If you are on the journey toward fitness, your own lifelong pilgrimage, you will lose fat and gain muscle. An obsession with weight is counterproductive. A woman, for example, may lose several inches from her waist and hips; in fact she may reshape her entire body and *gain* weight simply because muscle weighs more than fat. A rapid weight loss is unhealthy, even dangerous, and in the end will leave you with a fitness deficit (due to muscle loss and other factors).

"Our bodies are, to most of us, an inconvenient appendage to our head."

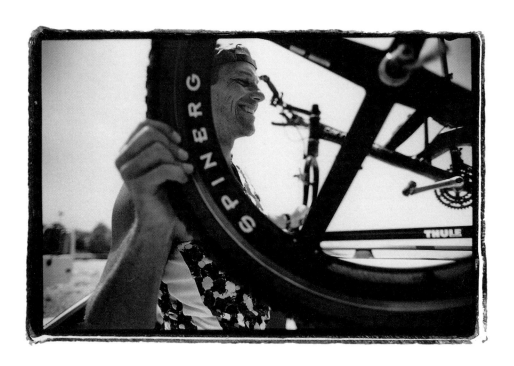

keeping in touch

The journey to fitness keeps
us in contact with nature.
The sights, smells, and
sounds of land and water
remind us of our relationship
to the material world.

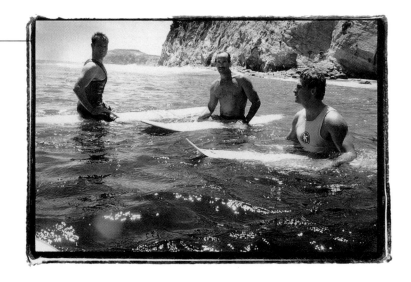

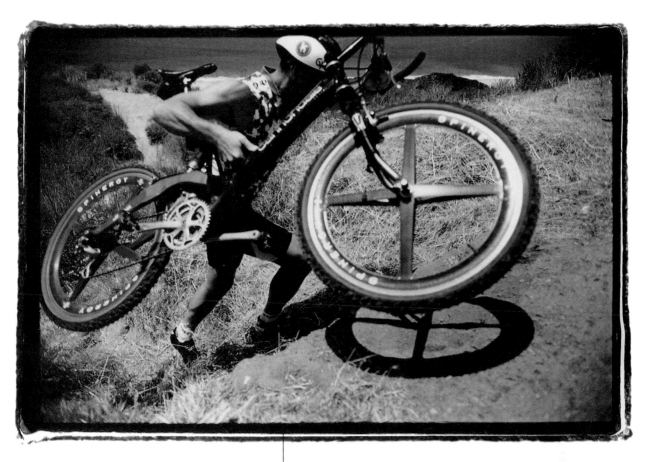

a sensory delight

The sound of your heart beating, the feel of muscles
working, and the smell of nature around you confirm your
existence as a living, breathing, physical being.

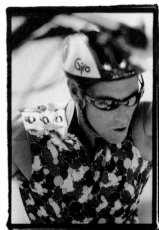

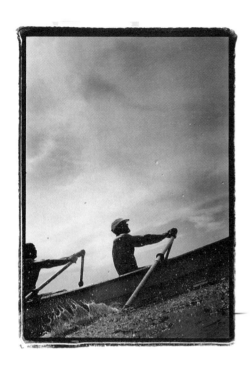

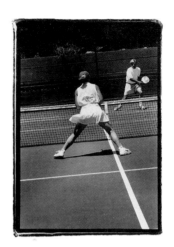

improved body chemistry

increased strength and muscle mass

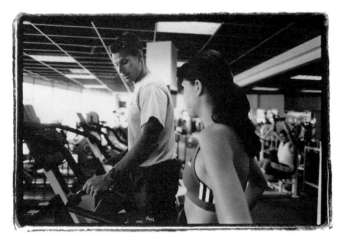

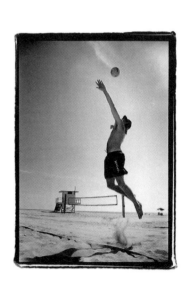

consistent weight control

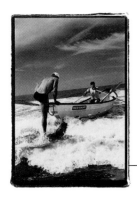

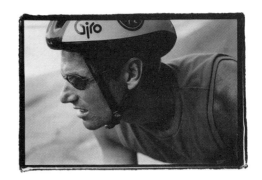

improved cardiovascular health

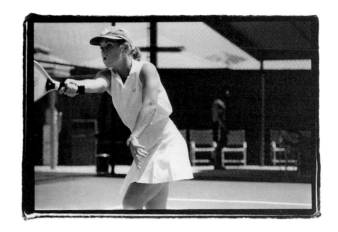

improved psychological health

improved quality of life

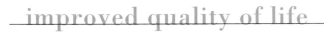

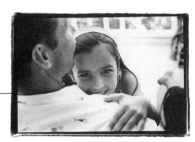

Many of us have an ingrained, deep-seated discomfort with our bodies. In this technological age we no longer do much physical work. Our bodies are, to most of us, an inconvenient appendage to our head. We make our living by reading, writing, speaking, and thinking, but seldom by physical labor.

Most of us are office workers, not construction workers, and consequently our muscles are atrophied from disuse. The nature of our work is written on our physiques, and the imprint of our sedentary lifestyles can be read in our posture, gait, and carriage. The physical profile of most middle-aged Americans is distressingly similar—necks canted forward, shoulders rounded, abdomens flaccid, appendages skinny and weak.

Our neglected bodies often serve only as a repository for stress, depression, and illness. Yet we seldom make the connection between our physical health and our mental and spiritual well-being. Our idea of stress relief is often a regimen of Prozac or the services of a clinical psychologist. While both of these approaches can be valid and sometimes necessary, why is it that we seldom seek to restore (or gain for the first time) a sense of inner peace through the pursuit of health and wholeness? Every one of my clients will tell you that their journey toward fitness has improved their sense of well-being, reduced their stress levels, and made them more productive.

"We have disassociated health from beauty and settled for a one-dimensional, impoverished concept."

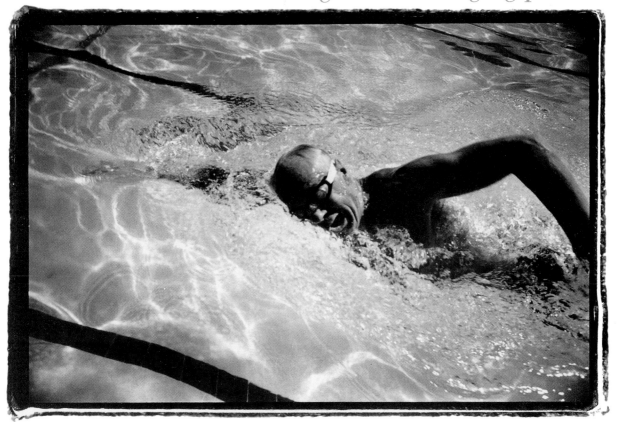

We live in our minds so much of the time that we have almost forgotten our bodies. To be sure, we admire some bodies for their superficial beauty. The human physique is publicly displayed more than at any other time in history. Yet in the midst of all the images of attractive young flesh many of us only feel detachment. We have disassociated health from beauty and settled for a one-dimensional, impoverished concept.

Beauty is part of a multi-dimensional reality, something you *live*. Real beauty is more than a perfectly posed, digitally retouched photo in a magazine or on a billboard. It is something we can all possess, because it is the end result of a whole and integrated person—body, mind, and spirit. We have lived too long with the mistaken idea that our physical, psychological, and spiritual health can be neatly separated. If you care for your body you will also nurture your mind and spirit. And if you care for your mind and spirit—truly care—you will nurture your body. In doing so, you will find true beauty, the kind that grows from the inside out.

"Exercise is like prayer—there's no reason to pray if you're not a believer."

This book contains a wide range of practical "how to" material, a little bit of scientific theory, and many examples of how my clients have adapted sound exercise and dietary principles into their individual lives. Since we all share certain common physiological traits, there are some basic things you need to know. However, as you work your way through the chapters that follow, constantly keep in mind that the most important element in a fit and healthy lifestyle is not technique, but attitude. You can know all the theory in the world, but if you do not have the right mindset, it will do you no good. Exercise is like prayer—there's no reason to pray if you're not a believer. You need to have faith before you can have a meaningful prayer life, and you must believe in the intrinsic value of health if you hope to achieve it. If you haven't seen the light, if you're not a convert, you will fail.

Thankfully, the benefits of becoming a convert are life changing. I can think of at least seven good reasons, but seven hardly exhaust the possibilities. If you are considering whether or not you should become a believer, here are some of the benefits of keeping the faith.

Seven Benefits of Keeping the Faith

- An improved quality of life
- A slowing down of the aging process
- Improved psychological health
- Consistent weight control
- Improved cardiovascular health
- Increased strength and muscle mass
- Improved body chemistry

Benefit 1: An Improved Quality of Life

It is too easy to think of fitness as an abstract set of statistics: blood pressure, body-fat percentage, weight. These numbers are useful and important, but those who keep the faith seldom think about them. They are too busy enjoying life! These people are particularly noticeable as they pass forty and begin to stand out from their peers—the majority of whom are unfit and unhealthy. I know and train people of all ages, some of whom have been on the journey of health for years. These people are really reaping the benefits of their good habits.

Regardless of your age, like the old man at Gold's Gym, you will be more energetic and enjoy a higher quality of life. You will be able to do physical things that most of your contemporaries will only be able to look on with envy, and you will have an attitude that will be an inspiration to everyone around you. People on the journey of fitness have a vitality and energy that is contagious.

Benefit 2: A Slowing Down of the Aging Process

I have clients in their seventies who are very fit and physically active. They have the strength, aerobic capacity, flexibility, and coordination of people decades younger. I have a sixty-year-old friend who surfs every weekend with his twenty-year-old son. In the winter he skis. I know men and women in their fifties who can hammer their mountain bikes up a ten-mile climb on a steep dirt road and leave eighteen-year-olds in their wake, gasping for breath. I know forty-year-old women who dance and practice yoga, who have the coordination and flexibility of teenage gymnasts.

All of these people are living proof that much of the physical incapacity we associate with age is avoidable and, in many cases, reversible. It is never too late or too early to begin the journey. If you are strong, flexible, and aerobically conditioned you will feel and look younger than your years. Physiological and calendar age are not the same.

Benefit 3: Improved Psychological Health

I know from long experience that exercise and healthy living build self-esteem and boost confidence in all aspects of my clients' personal and professional lives. They are less depressed, less anxious, less consumed by day-to-day pressures. A healthy lifestyle will pay many psychological dividends in ways that may surprise you. Exercise reduces the amount of adrenaline in the bloodstream and increases the amount of endorphins (a natural tranquilizer) produced by your body.

Many of my clients have reported an improvement in the quality of their sex lives, for example, because the positive attitudes they developed about their bodies translated into increased confidence in their sexual abilities. Other clients have reported a new sense of inner peace and calm, or the ability to control anger more effectively. The psychological benefits of exercise are unique to every person, but one thing is certain: Your mental outlook will improve.

Benefit 4: Consistent Weight Control

As we will see later, diets simply do not work. Diets leave you weak, dehydrated, and undernourished. A healthy lifestyle allows you to eat more, build strength, and ensure an adequate intake of vital nutrients. When you eat right and exercise, weight control is consistent and effortless. A healthy lifestyle ensures muscle growth and maintenance, stabilizes your blood sugar, encourages the production of fat-burning hormones, and increases your metabolism. A healthy lifestyle avoids the physically debilitating ups and downs of a typical weight-loss, weight-gain cycle.

For those who embrace fitness as a pilgrimage, weight maintenance is not a burden. When you commit to the journey for a lifetime, you can be easier on yourself in the short run. The road is much easier to traverse when it is a long, gradual climb. Dieting only dooms you to the fate of Sisyphus: an endless cycle of strenuous effort, followed by disheartening failure. When you exercise you can eat more, worry less, and forget about the privations of the latest fad diet.

Benefit 5: Improved Cardiovascular Health

A healthy lifestyle will drastically reduce your susceptibility to heart disease. If you reduce your intake of cholesterol, monitor your blood pressure, and avoid obesity, you will diminish your chances of suffering a heart attack, but you will not necessarily be healthy. Healthy people are active and enjoy life. And active people are far less likely to develop coronary heart disease, independent of any other factor. If you exercise aerobically you will multiply the benefits of a good diet, strengthen your coronary arteries, and have fun while doing it.

I counsel my clients to stop thinking about the specifics, lighten up, and play! People often focus on the burdensome aspects of avoiding heart disease: Don't eat certain foods, avoid stressful situations, get thirty minutes of exercise a day—or die! The advice always ends up sounding like John Calvin on a bad day—strict and austere. What will keep you going on the road to health is the satisfaction of doing something you enjoy. Good cardiovascular health will be the result of a program that comes from your figurative heart. You must love what you do. If you want to walk, run, dance, row, swim, cycle, in-line skate, cross-country ski, practice yoga—whatever—then *do* it. The joy of pursuing what you delight in will translate into a healthier heart.

Benefit 6: Increased Strength and Muscle Mass

Healthy people have good quality muscles. And what is a good quality muscle? In my opinion, it's not the kind you see on a stereotypical bodybuilder. Good quality muscles are what you see on an athlete. An athlete can *do* things with his or her body; their muscles are conditioned for performance, not size. And that's the point—good muscles literally empower you. Without them, you cannot perform the ordinary, everyday tasks of life, much less the extraordinary things of which healthy people are capable.

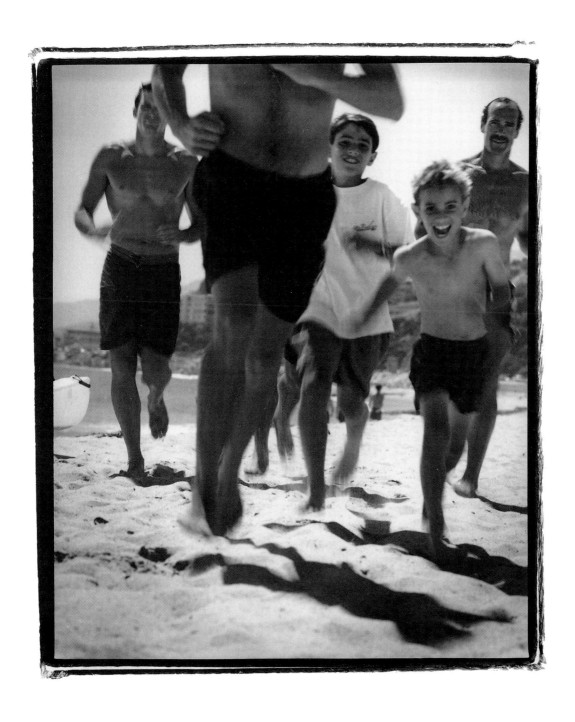

If you are young and your muscles are unconditioned, or if you are old and have let your muscles deteriorate, you have deprived yourself of the ability to perform at your peak—not only practical things, but fun things. When you are physically strong, a whole new world of possibilities opens up to you.

Healthy people have more muscle mass and less fat. This is good news if you like to eat. Muscle is much more metabolically active than fat—in other words, muscle burns more calories than fat, and it burns it twenty-four hours a day, seven days a week. This is one of the reasons fit people are able to control their weight. Every pound of muscle you gain increases your metabolism, so even when you're not exercising, you're burning more calories. And by the way, increased muscle mass will also improve bone density and mitigate the effects of osteoporosis in women. So if you trip and fall on the way to the buffet table, you're less likely to break a leg.

Benefit 7: Improved Body Chemistry

A healthy lifestyle will have a dramatic effect on what I loosely call "body chemistry." For example, when you exercise, your body produces a beneficial kind of cholesterol known as HDL. People who are active have significantly higher levels of HDL, a natural steroid that helps to clean your arteries of fatty plaque deposits (the bad cholesterol) that can contribute to heart disease, increased blood pressure, or strokes.

Regular exercise also changes the way your body processes an important hormone, insulin. This is good in two respects. First, people who are fit produce only about half the amount of insulin that sedentary people do. This greatly reduces the chance of developing adult-onset diabetes, an increasingly common disease in our overweight society. Second, when your body uses insulin more efficiently, it is able to process carbohydrates more efficiently, too, thus stabilizing your blood sugar. When your blood sugar is stable you are less likely to become hungry between meals, and you will have more energy.

Far too many Americans choose pain and disability rather than health. They have come to believe that the pursuit of health is a burden, an imposition on their already overscheduled, overcommitted lives. Yet, maintaining a healthy lifestyle is not burdensome—it is *liberating*. Time and money are of little worth without health. Success without vitality is of no value. It is never too late to get on the road. No matter what your age or physical condition, the time to begin is now.

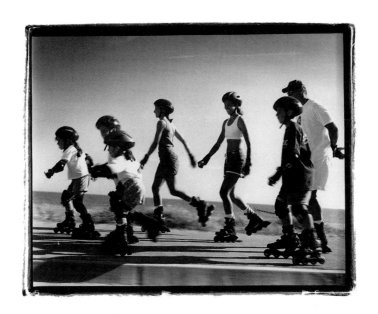

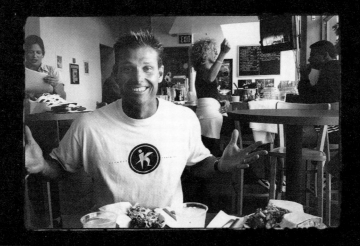

S P I R I T U A L F O O D

The turning point for me came one Saturday afternoon when I went to a matinee performance of the movie Jericho Mile. *In the movie, a prison inmate decides to become an Olympic-class runner, and in the process finds self-respect. The story and imagery of that film moved me in a deep place, and the following Monday I began my own quest for inner peace through the pursuit of fitness. I knew that nothing less than my own battered self-esteem was at stake. I could no longer live under the shadow of others' expectations. What I didn't realize was that my whole future would be changed by that decision. The coaches who had labeled me an under-achiever did not know what to make of my new found passion. There I was, with football season over, running hundreds of sets of stairs in the stadium after school. They had never been able to get me to do anything! What they didn't understand, was that I had made a decision for myself. To them, my new-found passion seemed to border on the fanatical. What had gotten in to me, they wondered? And I admit that I did have a sudden, surprising zeal for fitness. But it was not the zeal of a religious fanatic. It was the commitment of a disciple. I had found the faith.*

WHAT YOU EAT MATTERS

Many ancient religious traditions have made the connection between food, faith, and health. The dietary regulations of the Jews were an inseparable part of the Hebrew religion. Those same rules are maintained by many Jews today who only eat kosher foods. For them, maintaining a proper diet is an act of devotion. Historically, religions as diverse as those of Native Americans, Christian mystics, and Hindus have also advocated special dietary regimens. Religious people have widely believed that what they ate mattered and had a profound effect on them physically, psychologically, and spiritually.

"If fitness is religion then diet is a sacrament of the faith."

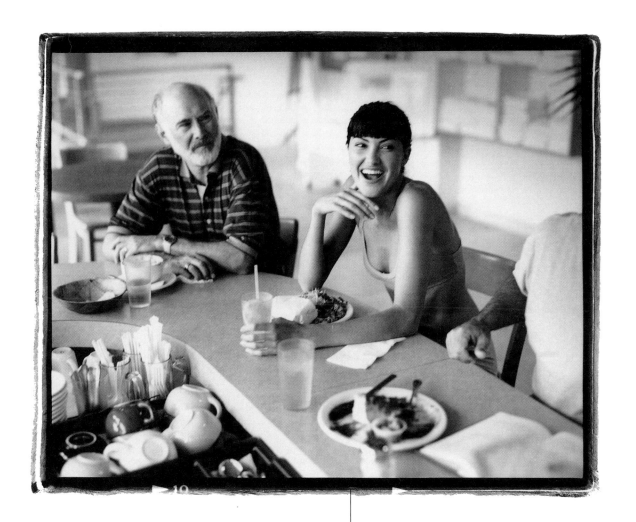

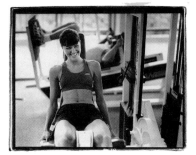

eat right, feel right

A healthy diet is the foundation on which a
healthy lifestyle is built. A good diet will
increase your energy, improve your
exercise program, reduce body fat, and
improve your cardiovascular health.

If fitness is religion then diet is a sacrament of the faith. In fact, good nutrition is the foundation on which a healthy lifestyle is built. A healthy diet will increase your energy; enhance your exercise program; reduce body fat; improve your sports performance; and decrease the odds of suffering from heart disease, hypertension, diabetes, and cancer. In other words, if you eat well, you will feel better, look better, perform better, and probably live longer! A good diet might even assist you in your spiritual development.

> "To be healthy we must keep in mind how God has created us or, if you prefer, how evolution has shaped us."

Human beings are amazingly adaptable when it comes to nutrition. We can survive on a wide variety of foods. But is survival the point? It seems to me that we should ask another question: What kind of diet do we need to thrive? I would suggest that to be healthy we must keep in mind how God has created us or, if you prefer, how evolution has shaped us. Whether you are a theist or an evolutionist, or both, the question is the same. How are we designed? What is the optimal diet given what we know about the physiology and chemistry of *Homo sapiens*? Could it be that our physical, psychological, and spiritual health are all shaped to some degree by what we eat? I believe so.

In 1986 two researchers published an article in the *New England Journal of Medicine* that suggested we may be genetically predisposed to eat certain kinds of foods. The article, now famous, gave birth to a concept that has come to be known as the caveman diet. The gist of the researchers' argument went something like this: Modern human beings appeared on earth about forty thousand years ago. Limited agriculture appeared about ten thousand years ago. Dietary habits now common in Western society began about a hundred years ago. Now what do you suppose people ate before the introduction of agriculture? Meat (protein). And lots of it. What happened after agriculture was developed, and our ancestors started eating mostly grains (carbohydrates)? They got weaker and smaller. The people who lived before the advent of farming were six inches taller than their descendants and had the bone density of Olympic athletes! What has happened in the last century? We have developed a whole panoply of ailments known as the "diseases of civilization."

"Were we genetically designed to eat certain kinds of foods, in certain proportions?"

Ancient peoples died from injuries and infectious diseases, but seldom from cancer or heart disease or hypertension. Now I'm not suggesting that you learn how to throw a spear and hunt "gregarious ungulate herbivores" as the researchers so eloquently describe what our ancestors ate (i.e., deer, bison, horses, etc.). What I am recommending, however, is that there is something to learn from their diet. The oldest humans, who appeared on earth several million years ago, and modern humans, who have been around for tens of thousands of years, consumed a lot of protein, fewer carbohydrates, less saturated fat, and more vitamins and minerals than we do. For most of our existence, we humans have rarely eaten grains, milk, or milk products. Is our modern diet out of sync with our physiology? Were we genetically designed to eat certain kinds of foods, in certain proportions? Perhaps so.

	Caveman Diet	Our Diet
Total Calories:		
Protein	34%	12%
Carbohydrates	45%	46%
Fat	21%	42%

As it turns out, the caveman diet looks something like the approach popularized by Dr. Barry Sears in his best-selling book, *The Zone*. Sears and others have recommended that we get about 40 percent of our calories from carbohydrates, 30 percent from protein, and 30 percent from fat. This is quite different from the prevailing advice we have been receiving from "experts" over the last decade. Most of them have been advising us to eat a low-fat, high complex-carbohydrate diet. And a lot of people have taken that advice. But guess what? As a nation we're fatter than ever before! All that pasta we've been eating has just ended up around our collective waist and hips. The high-carbohydrate diet has not worked. Why? The answer is very straightforward, and the facts have always been there for doctors and nutritionists to see. It's very basic science. Our physiology seems to have been optimized for a diet containing a certain amount of protein and fat. With insufficient protein and fat in our diet, we cannot achieve optimum health. Our genetic heritage won't be denied.

"A good diet simply recognizes and acknowledges the way we were designed and made."

All humans need six essential nutrients to live. These nutrients are carbohydrates, proteins, fats, vitamins, minerals, and water. Withhold any one of these long enough, and we die. Three of these essential nutrients are called "macro nutrients." We need macro nutrients in large quantities throughout the day because they are our main energy sources. Carbohydrates, protein, and fat are the macro nutrients. Vitamins, minerals, and water don't give us energy, although they are essential for our body to function. By the way, it's a mistake to think you can eat poorly and make up the difference by popping vitamin pills. Supplements are virtually useless without a good basic diet. If you want to live, you've got to have all the six essential nutrients. If you want to be *healthy*, you've got to get them in the right proportion. A good diet simply recognizes and supports the way we were designed and made.

The Six Essential Nutrients

Carbohydrates
Protein
Fat
Vitamins
Minerals
Water

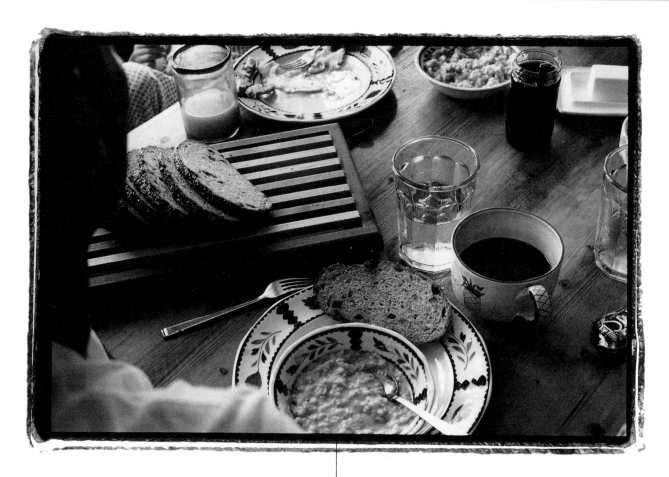

learn the principles

When you understand how proteins, fats, and carbohydrates are metabolized in your body, it's easy to design a program that is perfectly suited to your own particular lifestyle and needs.

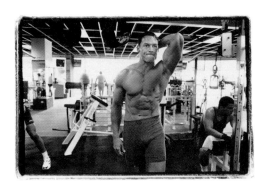

UNDERSTAND YOUR DIET
AND TAKE CONTROL

We've been taught for the last several years that the best diet is one high in complex carbohydrates and low in fat. I used to advocate that approach myself, but I've modified it somewhat. I've made a few changes in my own diet, and on the basis of the results I've experienced, I have recommended changes for my clients, too. Basically, I've reduced the amount of carbohydrates in my diet and have begun eating more protein and a little more fat. I was already pretty lean, but to my surprise, by making these changes and cutting down slightly on carbohydrates, I went from 11 percent body fat to less than 8 percent over a period of about two months. What became clear to me was that I had underestimated the fat building potential of consuming too many carbohydrates. I had also not realized the positive fat-loss benefits of consuming a certain quantity of dietary fat. It seemed counterintuitive to me that carbohydrates are so easily and routinely turned into fat. It certainly seemed odd that consuming a bit more dietary fat would help me to reduce my overall amount of body fat—but the results spoke for themselves.

"The people who keep the faith in the long run are those who understand the basis of their faith."

I try not to burden my clients with the minutiae of nutritional science. I think it's important to understand some basic principles of nutrition. If you understand the principles you're in a better position to make day-to-day decisions about what you eat and be aware of the consequences of ignoring your genetic heritage. Each of us has a unique set of genes, but

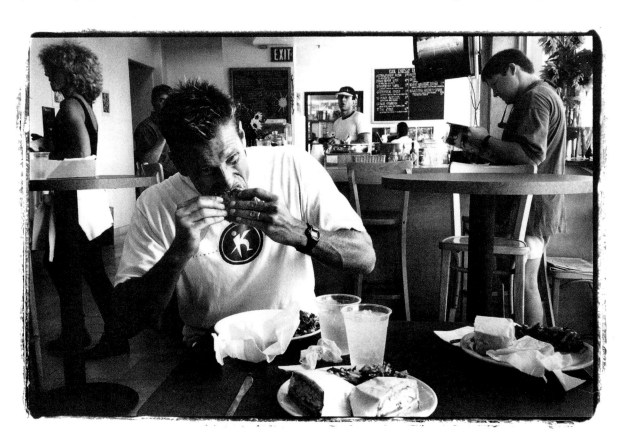

we all share some common physiological processes. If you understand something about those processes you can much more easily construct a diet and lifestyle that suits your own particular needs. The people who keep the faith in the long run are those who understand the basis of their faith. If you understand how your body processes the various kinds of foods you eat, then you are empowered to make decisions for yourself. So what are those processes? Let's start with the three macro nutrients and the role they play in meeting our body's nutritional needs. The first macro nutrient is carbohydrates.

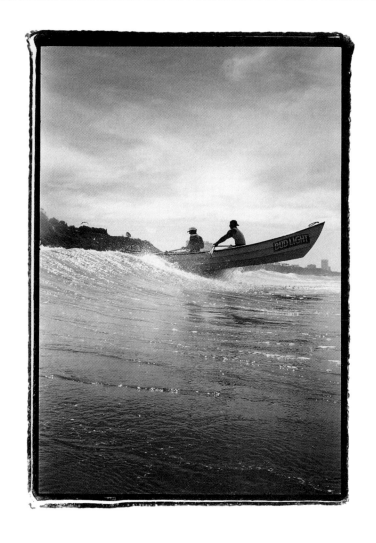

"Carbohydrate is merely the scientific name for sugar."

So what are carbohydrates? Simply put, they're sugar. Carbohydrate is merely the scientific name for sugar. Unfortunately, when we think of sugar, we imagine the white granulated stuff we add to our coffee or put in sweets, and little else. But an apple is sugar, too. Table sugar is a simple form of sugar, and an apple is a complex form of sugar—but in the end, in your bloodstream, they're both the same. Table sugar is a little chain made up of two molecules—a simple carbohydrate. When you eat table sugar it is quickly broken down and absorbed by your body because it has only two chemical links to break. The sugar from an apple, however, is a little more complicated—it's made up of more links—and therefore it takes your body longer to break it down into useable energy. Sugars with more links in their chain are called complex carbohydrates.

What About Vitamins?

If you are eating a healthy diet, you will be getting most of the vitamins you need. Nevertheless, I recommend that you take a good quality multi-vitamin and mineral supplement. A good supplement will help fill in the gaps in your diet and provide sufficient quantities of vital minerals that are often missing in processed foods.

In general, complex carbohydrates are better for you because they break down more slowly in your body and give you more long-term energy. But there's more. Complex carbohydrates—vegetables for example—are also high in fiber. Fiber slows down the conversion of carbohydrates into blood sugar. Blood sugar, which is called glucose, is stored in the body in the form of a substance called glycogen, and glycogen is one of your body's sources of energy. But the trick is not to get too much glucose in your blood all at once. Your body makes a hormone called insulin to transport glucose into storage. Insulin works to store a small quantity of glucose as glycogen in your muscles, a larger quantity in your liver, and the rest in a place you might not expect.

"You can eat a completely fat-free diet and still be grossly overweight."

If you have more glucose in your blood than you can store in your muscles and liver, insulin works to put the excess in storage somewhere else—your fat cells. Your body can only store away enough glycogen in your muscles and liver for about two hours worth of energy. After that, everything else goes into storage as *fat*. All those extra carbohydrates you've been eating are still hanging around—literally. They've been converted into body fat. A simple analogy helps me remember how this process works. Think of your body as having two fuel tanks, a little one and a big one. The little one is your liver. It fills up quickly. Once your liver is full, the insulin will take that glucose and store it away as fat. Fat is the big fuel tank. And that big fuel tank has an unlimited capacity.

Not surprisingly, you can eat a completely fat-free diet and still be grossly overweight. Because of all the talk about fat-free diets, however, we've come to think that dietary fat equals body fat, and therefore if we avoid eating fat, we won't get fat. This is a mistake many dietitians and nutritionists have been making for a long time. What we've overlooked is the fact that insulin is not only a storage hormone, it's a fat-making hormone, too. This is true not only for humans, but for animals. Cows eat an all-carbohydrate diet of grains and molasses. They don't eat any meat or ice cream. Cows are fattened up for market by consuming a fat-free diet!

"That lull in energy that many of us feel in between meals is the result of a drop in our blood sugar."

A so-called healthy diet of carbohydrates can cause real problems for us in our daily lives. We can become carbo junkies. Carbohydrates are the brain's main energy source. The brain needs almost no fat or protein; it's fueled by glucose. Consequently, people who eat too many carbohydrates can set themselves up for trouble. Let's say that you eat a "healthy" breakfast at eight o'clock in the morning consisting of cereal with skim milk, a piece of fruit, a glass of orange juice, and black coffee. This

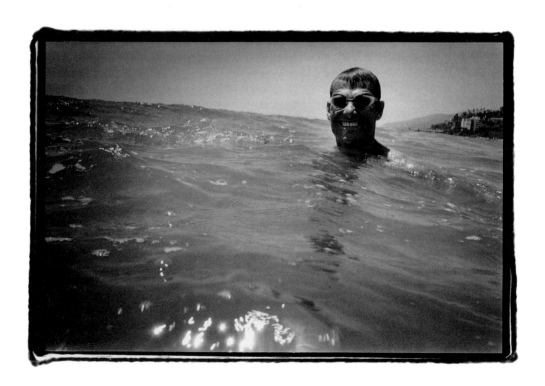

breakfast is almost all carbohydrates, has virtually no fat, and very little protein. By ten o'clock you're feeling a lull in your energy. Why? All those carbohydrates were converted into glucose, which made your blood sugar rise dramatically. The glucose stimulated the production of insulin. The insulin rushed to the bloodstream and did its job of transporting the glucose into storage, and then your blood sugar dropped. Your brain, which runs on glucose, said, "Send me some more glucose!" You're suddenly consumed by the need to eat something sweet. You take out a plastic container full of sliced peaches and pears—more healthy food. Your blood sugar rises and you're satisfied for another couple of hours. But by lunch you're starving again. You go to lunch and head for the pasta bar. You load up on high-carbohydrate food. Temporarily you're full. You go back to the office, but by two o'clock you're starving again.

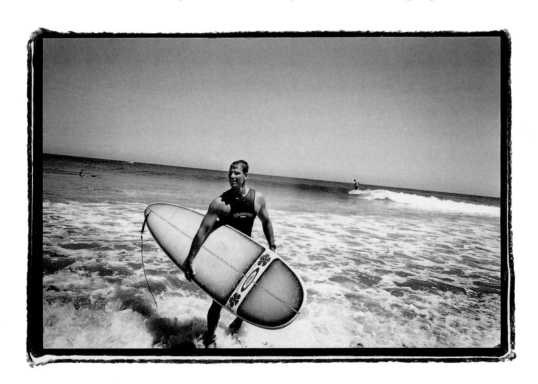

Carbohydrates—The Best and The Worst

Favorable (Stimulate the Least Insulin)
Barley, oatmeal, rye, apples, pears, grapes, grapefruit, peaches, kidney beans, lima beans, soy beans, peas, peanuts, milk, and yogurt

Unfavorable (Stimulate the Most Insulin)
Processed grains (including most bread), corn chips, simple sugars, commercial cereals, carrots, corn, bananas, raisins, apricots, low-fat ice cream (if you're going to sin, sin boldly)

This scenario is familiar to many of us who have tried a diet consisting mostly of carbohydrates. The phenomenon is called blood-sugar yo-yoing. That lull in energy that many of us feel in between meals is the result of a drop in our blood sugar. When we eat a high-carbohydrate diet and don't get enough protein and fat, we end up establishing a rising-falling cycle of our blood glucose levels that stimulates the brain to want more and more carbohydrates. In effect, we are teaching our bodies to crave and burn sugar. The only way to stop this cycle is to manage our insulin levels, and one of the ways we can accomplish this is to balance our consumption of carbohydrates with some protein and fat.

"You may look the same from day to day but your body is always rebuilding and renewing itself."

Proteins, or the amino acids from them, are the building blocks of life.

The most common use of protein is the rebuilding of our body's tissues. Protein is also essential for the functioning of our nervous system, for growth, and for the production of vital enzymes, antibodies, and hormones. There are twenty-two components, or amino acids, in protein, and ten of them are called "essential" because we must get them from the food we eat. These amino acids are, quite literally, building blocks. The human body is an amazing thing. It is always in a state of flux. For example, every seven years we have completely new skin. The oldest red blood cell in our body is only about 120 days old. Every three days the walls of our intestines are completely new. You may look the same from day to day but your body is always rebuilding and renewing itself. Protein plays a vital role in this on-going process of rejuvenation.

Protein Sources—The Best and The Worst

Favorable (Low Fat)
Chicken breast, turkey breast, lean pork, liver, extra-lean beef, water-pack tuna, salmon, halibut, cod, egg whites, tofu, protein powder, low-fat or no-fat cottage cheese

Unfavorable (High Fat)
Bacon, most beef, pepperoni, most sausages, salami, most hot dogs, hard cheeses

Protein also plays a key role in regulating blood sugar and helping your body to metabolize fat. Protein, like carbohydrates, is responsible for stimulating the production of another important hormone in our body. Whereas carbohydrates stimulate the production of insulin, which stores energy, protein stimulates the production of a substance called glucagon. Glucagon is called a mobilization hormone, because it moves energy out of storage and puts it to work. Insulin and glucagon work together like a seesaw. When one goes up, the other goes down. Insulin stores energy in our fuel tanks, and glucagon helps to empty the tank. Glucagon is also known as a fat mobilizing hormone because it will go to the big fuel tank, our fat reserves, and release the caloric energy stored there. If you are eating too many carbohydrates your blood insulin levels will be high, and your glucagon level will be low. You can't burn much fat if your glucagon levels are suppressed.

"If it were possible for you to eliminate all fat from your diet you'd be dead in about six weeks."

In addition to carbohydrates and protein, fat is an essential food source, too. Without fat, you'll die. If it were possible for you to eliminate all fat from your diet you'd be dead in about six weeks. Fortunately, this is not really possible. As we've seen, our wonderfully adaptive bodies can make fat out of carbohydrates. So what does fat do for us except make us jiggle? Fat cushions our vital organs, insulates our bodies, stores energy, and helps us to utilize certain vitamins. Fat also helps us to produce a hormone, called CCK, that sends a signal to the brain that says, "Stop! I'm full." That's why fats satisfy our hunger longer. And fat performs another beneficial function—it slows down the conversion of carbohydrates into glucose. Fat, like protein, helps to stabilize our blood sugar.

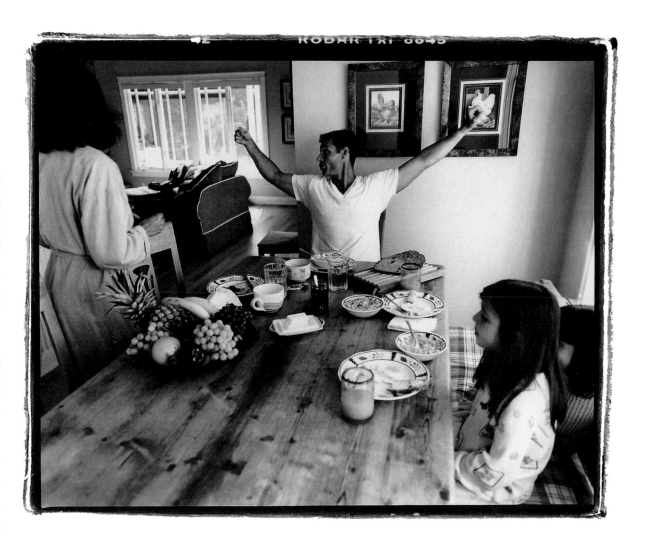

"Food, just like prescription drugs, affects the body's hormones in profound ways."

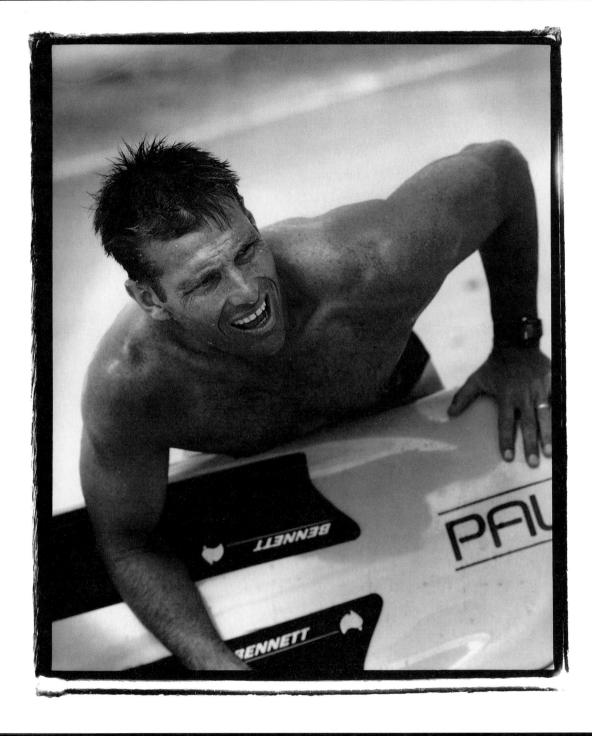

Fat is a very concentrated form of energy. A gram of fat has about nine calories, whereas a gram of carbohydrate or protein has only about four calories. It doesn't take much fat on our bodies to provide huge reserves of caloric energy. An elite athlete, like a marathoner, might have body fat as low as 4 percent. But even at 4 percent, that marathoner will probably have in the range of 50,000 calories' worth of body fat. That's enough to run about twenty marathons, back to back. On the other hand, that same marathoner will have only about two hours' worth of energy stored away in his liver. Just because he's an elite athlete doesn't mean he has a bigger sugar tank. The most successful endurance athletes today are putting more protein and fat in their diets, because it helps them to more readily access their fat reserves. This helps them avoid "hitting the wall" when they deplete their liver of glycogen.

Fat Sources—The Best and The Worst

Favorable (High in Monounsaturated Fat)
Olive oil, canola oil, peanut oil, almond butter, peanut butter (the natural kind)

Okay in Moderation (Low in Saturated Fat)
Light mayonnaise, sesame oil, soybean oil

Unfavorable (High in Saturated Fat)
Shortening, lard, butter, cream, sour cream, cream cheese, hydrogenated and partially hydrogenated oils (butter substitutes)

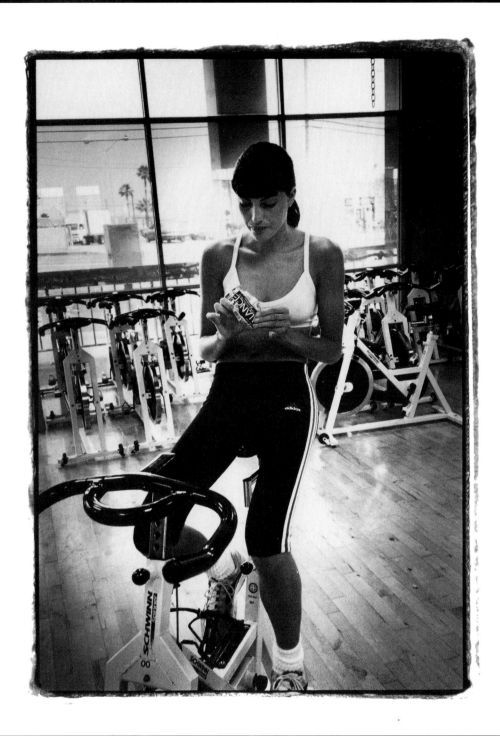

FOOD IS A DRUG
USE IT WISELY

Food, just like prescription drugs, affects the body's hormones in profound ways. As we have seen, carbohydrates, protein, and fat all stimulate different hormones. The goal of a healthy diet is to find a balance that works with your body's natural processes to provide good energy, stabilize blood sugar, and burn fat. A sensible diet can do all of this without resorting to the extreme measures of liquid protein diets, high-carbohydrate diets, or any of the other fads that make the headlines weekly. My own experience indicates that a diet of approximately 40 percent carbohydrates, 30 percent protein, and 30 percent fat works well for many people. But I'm not legalistic about that ratio. I think it's a good reference point, a place to start. The 40–30–30 approach seems to provide a good equilibrium between the brain's need to have enough glucose, the body's need to repair and build itself, and the benefits of a certain amount of dietary fat. I would encourage you to experiment. Some people require more protein, others less fat. Strive for a balance that works for you and eat experimentally. Pay attention to what you consume and how it affects the way you feel.

"What you eat determines whether you are going to burn fat or store it."

Fortunately, a balanced diet turns out to be what most of us would consider a fairly normal meal. You don't have to suffer. You don't have to count every calorie. To illustrate this, I like to use the example of a deli sandwich of sliced turkey on rye. A typical sandwich will have about four ounces of meat. An ounce of lean meat will have on average about 7 grams of protein and 3 grams of fat (or less). Two slices of bread will have about 30 grams of carbohydrates. When you add in low-fat mayo, pickles, tomato, mustard, and lettuce, you come out with about 28 grams of protein, 40 grams of carbohydrates, and 12 grams of fat. Converted into calories, this meal would be approximately 35 percent carbohydrates, 33 percent protein, and 32 percent fat. This is a healthy ratio and not far from the target of 40–30–30.

What about an alternative light breakfast, a low-calorie substitute for the high-carbohydrate "healthy" breakfast I mentioned earlier? Try a slice of whole-wheat bread and two egg whites with one yolk. This breakfast is barely more than 250 calories, but it is balanced. It has carbohydrates (the bread), protein (the egg whites), and fat (the yolk). This will satisfy you longer than an all-carbohydrate breakfast of 500 calories. If you have average metabolism, in the period between breakfast and lunch your body might expend 400 to 500 calories. With a

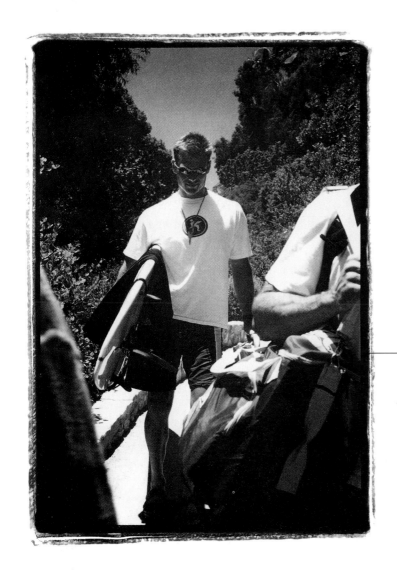

"A healthy diet has the potential to affect every aspect of our being—body, mind, and spirit."

balanced diet, however, 200 to 250 of those calories can come from stored fat. A balanced meal will help keep your insulin-glucagon levels in a favorable balance. You'll feel better and be less hungry between meals. It's surprising, but true: What you eat can determine whether you are going to burn fat or store it.

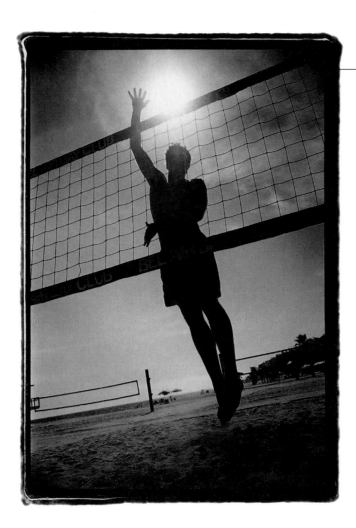

breakfast of champs

A healthy breakfast provides the energy you need to be active and energetic throughout the morning. Skip breakfast and your blood sugar will plummet.

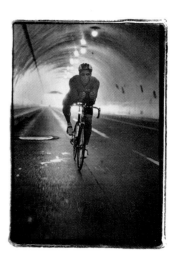

eat to win

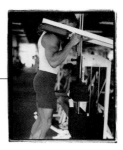

You can't build and repair muscles without sufficient protein in your diet. If you're working hard but not making progress, consider upping your protein intake.

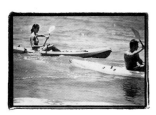

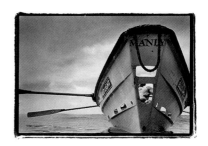

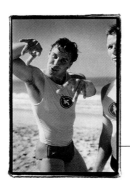

attitude is everything

A good diet is the result of a good attitude. If you value health, you'll want to eat well. When you make the connection between feeling well and eating well, a good diet is never a burden.

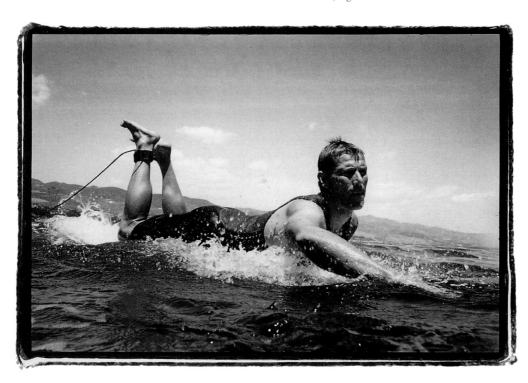

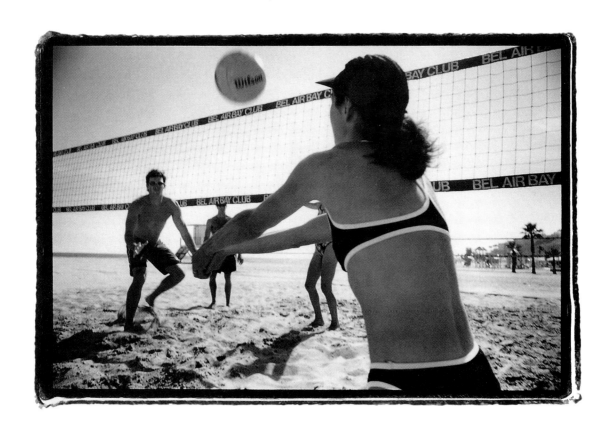

energy

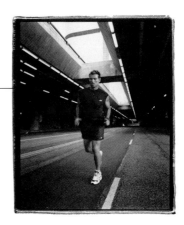

Good energy depends on
maintaining stable blood sugar
levels. A balanced diet, one
that includes sufficient fat and
protein, will help maintain
energy throughout the day.

I said at the beginning of this chapter that what you eat will have an effect on you physically, psychologically, and spiritually. I think this is true in part because we were designed with certain physiological traits. There are consequences that result from the decision to ignore the body's basic predispositions. The physical consequences are obvious—obesity, heart disease, diabetes, hypertension, cancer—but the psychological and spiritual consequences are real as well. Your mental state is profoundly affected by blood sugar levels. You will think more clearly and avoid mental fatigue if you stabilize your insulin levels by eating a balanced diet. And your spiritual self? If, as several of the world's religions affirm, the body is the temple of the spirit, how can our spirits thrive if the temple is in disrepair? Food is the raw material of which our bodies are made and maintained. Consequently, a healthy diet has the potential to affect every aspect of our being—body, mind, and spirit.

Fast Food—A Nutritional Analysis

	Calories	Protein	Fat	Carbs
Big Mac (with fries and shake)	1,100	40g	41g	143g
Whopper (with fries and shake)	1,200	40g	47g	147g
Pizza Hut (10" cheese pizza)	1,025	65g	23g	140g
Kentucky Fried Chicken (3-piece dinner)	1,000	55g	55g	71g

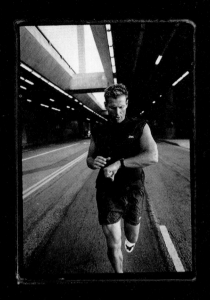

PRACTICAL MATTERS

A few weeks after I decided to get on the road to fitness, I scraped together thirty dollars and joined a local gym. I found myself getting fit and strong there, gaining confidence and finding my place in the world. Outside the gym, I assembled a library of books and magazines on health and fitness. I needed to know and experience everything. I wanted to get the most from my workouts. I even considered becoming a competitive bodybuilder. Soon, I decided to change gyms—to join a more "serious" place. The best facility in my area was the legendary Gold's Gym, in Santa Monica. I got a job there as manager. Gold's Gym was an astounding place, a veritable human menagerie. There were monstrously big, extreme bodybuilders, and there were ordinary people. And everything in between. But the ordinary folks, as a rule, did not aspire to look like the extreme bodybuilders. They wanted to look more like me. I had quickly given up my aspirations to be a competitive bodybuilder in favor of a more athletic but still muscular look. People began to ask me for training advice. I started helping them informally.

THE GOAL IS BALANCE

In the last chapter we talked about some of the philosophical and physiological aspects of nutrition. In this chapter we're going to look at nutrition from a practical perspective. We've already learned that the proportion of protein, carbohydrates, and fat in our diet is a key to maintaining stable blood sugar levels and improving our body's ability to metabolize fat. But exactly how do we put that insight into action? One of the most important things you can do is begin to add protein to every meal and snack you eat. Ultimately, I don't want you to worry too much about figuring out if you are getting the "optimum" ratio of 40 percent carbohydrates, 30 percent protein, and 30 percent fat. I consider those percentages to be a guideline and not a strict rule. Since most Americans eat too many carbohydrates, replacing a percentage of them with protein is the logical place to start.

What I want you to do for a while is pay close attention to what you eat, overcome old bad habits, and learn to consume a balanced diet. The so-called healthy breakfast I mentioned in the last chapter is a good example of a bad habit. If you're eating only cereal and fruit in the morning, be aware that you are eating almost all carbohydrates. Add some protein. As you observe and learn, you will gradually develop an

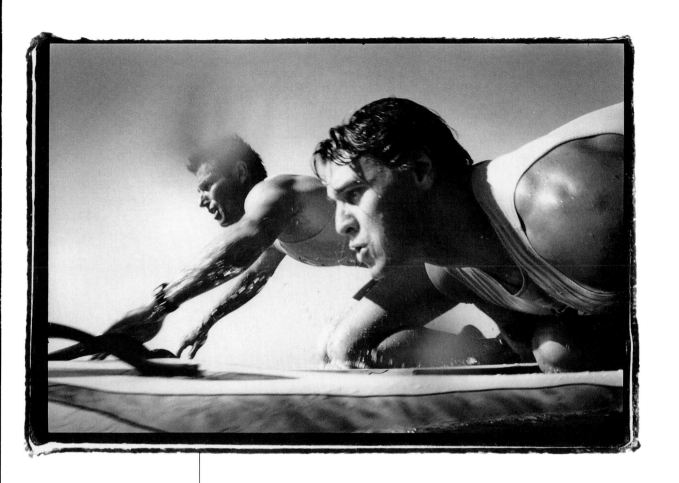

burning calories

A good diet is no substitute for exercise. It makes no sense to eat
well while pursuing a sedentary lifestyle. Exercise increases
metabolism and burns more calories. When you are fit, your
body utilizes nutrients more effectively.

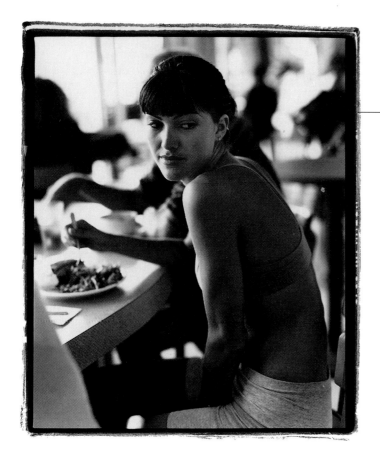

Your body quickly adapts when you don't eat enough, and lowers its metabolism. By eating too little, you set yourself up for future weight gains.

intuition for the ratio of nutrients you consume. After a while, you will know if you have the ratio right by the way you *feel*. If your blood sugar is stable and your insulin-glucagon levels are in balance, you will feel better, have more energy, and be less drowsy.

Whether you are just beginning the journey of fitness or you are a seasoned athlete, there are some general nutritional guidelines you should always keep in mind. Even if you decide not to follow the program that follows, these simple rules will make a significant difference in your health.

Don't be obsessed with weight.

It's the ratio of lean body mass (bones, internal organs, and muscle) to fat that counts. If you are tracking your weight, however, weigh yourself only once a week, on the same day. Your weight will vary from day to day largely on the basis of how much water is in your system.

Don't skip meals.

Skipping meals will only play havoc with your blood sugar levels and program your metabolism to store more fat. You may also lose muscle tissue and lower your basal metabolism.

Keep yourself well hydrated.

Most adults should drink at least eight glasses of water per day. When you are dehydrated, your body stores more water, not less. After a few days of sufficient hydration, your body will not hold as much water.

Don't consume more than about 600 calories per meal if you are trying to lose weight.

This is the maximum number of calories that most people can metabolize without storing fat. Eat smaller meals and supplement with healthy snacks.

Don't consume too much caffeine.

Caffeine will cause a slight rise in your blood insulin level. A little bit is okay, but use restraint.

Make sure the fats you consume are healthy.

Olive oil and canola oil are best for cooking and salad dressings.

Read labels.

Many processed foods contain hydrogenated fats and oils. Avoid foods like crackers, cookies, tortillas, etc. Hydrogenated oils are bad for your health.

Avoid saturated fats.

Try to limit your consumption of saturated fats to no more than 10 percent of your fat intake.

Use low-fat sources of protein.

Chicken and turkey white meat, fish, low-fat or no-fat cottage cheese, and tofu are excellent sources.

Use 1% or nonfat milk.

The difference in fat content between 1% and 2% low-fat is roughly equivalent to a pat of butter per glass.

Just adding a little protein to every meal will make a difference for many people, but a more precise and scientific way to determine your own nutritional requirement is to estimate the amount of protein you need based on three variables: your activity level, percentage of body fat, and weight. Use the workup sheet on page 80 to make your own calculations based on these variables.

I've filled out two sample workups so you can see how the calculations are made. The sample workup sheets are for a hypothetical man who is very physically active, but wants to shed that last stubborn pound or two of fat around his waist, and for a woman who is moderately active, but wants to shed fat without losing corresponding muscle tissue. I've included a blank workup sheet for you to photocopy and fill out for yourself. The calculation from your workup sheet will result in your daily protein requirement (DPR), a useful number that will allow you to make further calculations and determine some basic dietary guidelines for yourself. The guidelines (the overall number of calories you should consume, plus the amounts of protein, carbohydrates, and fat) are keyed to sample menus that follow.

Additionally, I've included tables to help you determine your body fat percentage. These tables will give you an approximation only, not an exact measure. If you belong to a health club and have access to a more accurate means of determining your body fat (a caliper test or flotation tank), you should use those methods. Finally, remember that all these calculations, and the dietary recommendations based on them, are meant to be a *learning tool,* not a way of life. I want you to develop an intuitive feel for what you eat, its nutritional content, and its effect on your body. Once you've learned how to eat, I want you to relax and forget about counting calories and grams.

Bio-Foods, makers of the Balance nutrition bar, has developed a comprehensive nutritional program described in their booklet *Better Health with Balance*. The following Personal Workup Sheet, calculation method, body fat tables, Meal Planning Guides, and menu guidelines are reproduced here with their permission.

PERSONAL WORKUP SHEET

NAME: JOHN SMITH   DATE: 11/97   HEIGHT: 6'1"   WEIGHT: 180

ACTIVITY FACTOR VARIABLES

0.5	Sedentary—no exercise
0.6	Light training/walking/jogging
0.7	Moderate aerobic training 3 times per week
0.8	Daily aerobic activity/light weight training
0.9	Heavy training 5 times per week
1.0	Heavy daily or twice daily training

0.2	Add if you stand at work for long periods
0.2	Add if you do strenuous work
1+	Add 0.1 for every hour above two hours hard training

CALCULATION

1. Enter your activity variable here.   .95
2. Enter your estimated body fat percentage here.   11%
   If you don't know your body fat percentage, use the table on page 87.
3. Enter your total body weight.   180
4. Multiply line 2 by line 3. (.11 x 180) This is your body fat in pounds.   20
5. Subtract line 4 from 3. This is your lean body mass.   160
6. Enter your activity factor from the variables above.   .95
7. Multiply line 5 by your activity factor. This is your
   estimated daily protein requirement in grams (DPR).   152

PERSONAL WORKUP SHEET

NAME: MARY SMITH   DATE: 11/97   HEIGHT: 5'7"   WEIGHT: 135

ACTIVITY FACTOR VARIABLES

0.5	Sedentary—no exercise
0.6	Light training/walking/jogging
0.7	Moderate aerobic training 3 times per week
0.8	Daily aerobic activity/light weight training
0.9	Heavy training 5 times per week
1.0	Heavy daily or twice daily training

0.1	Add if nursing
0.2	Add if you stand at work for long periods
0.2	Add if you do strenuous work
1+	Add 0.1 for every hour above two hours hard training

CALCULATION

1. Enter your activity variable here.   .7

2. Enter your estimated body fat percentage here.   23%
   If you don't know your body fat percentage, use the table on page 89.

3. Enter your total body weight. 135

4. Multiply line 2 by line 3. (.23 x 135) This is your body fat in pounds.   31

5. Subtract line 4 from 3. This is your lean body mass. 104

6. Enter your activity factor from the variables above. .7

7. Multiply line 5 by your activity factor. This is your
   estimated daily protein requirement in grams (DPR).   73*

*Do not go below 76 grams of protein per day—this is the minimum, so Mary should round up to 76.

PERSONAL WORKUP SHEET

NAME:　　　　　**DATE:**　　　　　**HEIGHT:**　　　　　**WEIGHT:**

ACTIVITY FACTOR VARIABLES

0.5	Sedentary—no exercise	
0.6	Light training/walking/jogging	
0.7	Moderate aerobic training 3 times per week	
0.8	Daily aerobic activity/light weight training	
0.9	Heavy training 5 times per week	
1.0	Heavy daily or twice daily training	
0.1	Add if nursing	
0.2	Add if you stand at work for long periods	
0.2	Add if you do strenuous work	
1+	Add 0.1 for every hour above two hours hard training	

CALCULATION

1.	Enter your activity variable here.	
2.	Enter your estimated body fat percentage here. If you don't know your body fat percentage, use the tables on pages 87 and 89.	
3.	Enter your total body weight.	
4.	Multiply line 2 by line 3. This is your body fat in pounds.	
5.	Subtract line 4 from 3. This is your lean body mass.	
6.	Enter your activity factor from the variables above.	
7.	Multiply line 5 by your activity factor. This is your estimated daily protein requirement in grams (DPR).	

(Photocopy this page for your own personal use.)

Once you have estimated your protein requirement in grams, you can extrapolate the approximate number of calories your body needs per day, including carbohydrates and fats, by a simple process of multiplication.

CALCULATING YOUR TOTAL DAILY REQUIREMENT
In Calories and Carbohydrate Grams

Calculation 1

Take your daily protein requirement (DPR) and multiply it by 13.33. This is the total number of calories from all food sources you need per day.

Example 1 (Joe Smith)

(Joe's DPR) 152 x 13.33 = 2,026 calories.
Total caloric need for Joe Smith is 2,026 calories per day.

Example 2 (Mary Smith)

(Mary's DPR) 76 x 13.33 = 1,013 calories.
Total caloric need for Mary Smith is 1,013 calories per day.

(My DPR) _____ x 13.33 = _____ my total daily caloric need.

Calculation 2

Multiply your daily protein requirement (DPR) by 4. This will tell you how many calories from protein you need per day.

Example 1 (Joe Smith)

(Joe's DPR) 152 x 4 = 608 calories.
Total protein calories per day is 608.

Example 1 (Mary Smith)

(Mary's DPR) 76 x 4 = 304 calories.
Total protein calories per day is 304.
(My DPR) _____ x 4 = _____ my daily protein need in calories.

Calculation 3

Multiply your daily protein requirement (DPR) by 1.33. This will tell you how many grams of carbohydrates you need per day.

Example 1 (Joe Smith)

(Joe's DPR) 152 x 1.33 = 202
Total carbohydrate grams per day is 202.

Example 2 (Mary Smith)

(Mary's DPR) 76 x 1.33 = 101
Total carbohydrate grams per day is 101.

(My DPR) _____ x 1.33 = my daily carbohydrate need in grams.

Calculation 4

Multiply your daily protein requirement (DPR) by 5.33. This will tell you how many calories from carbohydrates you need per day.

Example 1 (Joe Smith)

(Joe's DPR) 152 x 5.33 = 809
Total carbohydrate calories per day is 809.

Example 2 (Mary Smith)

(Mary's DPR) 76 x 5.33 = 405
Total carbohydrate calories per day is 405.
(My DPR) _____ x 5.33 = my daily carbohydrate need in calories.

Calculation 5

Multiply your daily protein requirement (DPR) by .44. This will tell you how many <u>grams of fat</u> you need per day.

Example 1 (Joe Smith)

(Joe's DPR) 152 x .44 = 67
Total fat grams per day is 67.

Example 2 (Mary Smith)

(Mary's DPR) 76 x .44 = 33.3
Total fat grams per day is 33.3.

(My DPR) _____ x .44 = my daily fat need in grams.

Calculation 6

Multiply your daily protein requirement (DPR) by 4. This will tell you how many <u>calories from fat</u> you need per day.

Example 1 (Joe Smith)

(Joe's DPR) 152 x 4 = 608 calories.
Total fat calories per day is 608 .

Example 1 (Mary Smith)

(Mary's DPR) 76 x 4 = 304 calories.
Total fat calories per day is 304.

(My DPR) _____ x 4 = my daily fat need in calories.

WORKUP SHEET SUMMARY

(Fill in the Results of Your Calculations)

Total Nutritional Need:

_____ calories per day (from Calculation 1)

Protein:

_____ grams of protein (DPR from Workup Sheet)
_____ calories from protein (from Calculation 2)

Carbohydrates:

_____ grams of carbohydrates (from Calculation 3)
_____ calories from carbohydrates (from Calculation 4)

Fat:

_____ grams of fat (from Calculation 5)
_____ calories from fat (from Calculation 6)

DAILY RECORD

(Keep a Record of Your Daily Consumption)

	Protein Grams	Carbohydrate Grams	Fat Grams
Breakfast			
Snack			
Lunch			
Snack			
Dinner			
Snack			
TOTAL			

(Photocopy this page for your own personal use.)

Body Fat Percentages for Men

TABLE 1

For Average Males Who Exercise Moderately 3 Times Per Week
(If Non-Exerciser Add 2%)

HEIGHT	WEIGHT										
	150	160	170	180	190	200	210	220	230	240	250
5'6"	17	19	21	23	25	27	29	31	33	35	37
5'7"	16	18	20	22	24	26	28	30	31	33	35
5'8"	14	15	18	20	22	24	26	28	30	32	33
5'9"	12	14	16	18	20	22	24	26	28	30	32
5'10"	10	12	13	16	18	20	22	24	26	28	30
5'11"	9	11	13	15	17	19	20	22	24	26	28
6'	8	9	11	13	15	17	19	20	22	24	26
6'1"	8	9	10	12	14	16	18	19	20	22	24
6'2"	-	7	9	11	13	15	17	19	21	22	23
6'3"	-	-	8	10	12	14	16	18	20	21	22
6'4"	-	-	7	9	11	13	15	17	19	20	21

TABLE 2
For Average Males Who Exercise Daily
(Including Aerobics and Resistance Training)

WEIGHT											
HEIGHT	150	160	170	180	190	200	210	220	230	240	250
5'6"	15	17	19	20	22	24	26	28	30	32	34
5'7"	14	16	18	20	22	24	26	28	30	31	33
5'8"	12	14	16	18	20	22	24	26	28	30	32
5'9"	10	13	15	16	18	20	22	24	26	28	30
5'10"	8	10	13	14	15	17	20	23	25	27	29
5'11"	7	9	12	13	14	16	18	20	22	24	26
6'	5	8	10	12	13	15	17	19	21	23	25
6'1"	5	7	9	11	12	14	16	18	20	22	24
6'2"	-	5	7	9	11	13	15	17	19	21	23
6'3"	-	-	6	8	10	12	14	15	17	19	21
6'4"	-	-	5	7	9	11	13	14	15	17	19

Body Fat Percentages for Women

TABLE 3

For Average Females Who Exercise Moderately 3 Times Per Week
(If Non-Exerciser Add 3%)

HEIGHT	WEIGHT										
	100	110	120	130	140	150	160	170	180	190	200
5'	23	26	29	36	40	44	46	48	50	50	50
5'1"	21	24	26	34	38	40	44	46	49	50	50
5'2"	18	20	26	32	35	39	42	46	49	50	50
5'3"	17	22	25	32	33	36	40	43	46	49	50
5'4"	16	26	28	30	31	32	34	36	38	42	46
5'5"	-	20	26	28	30	32	34	36	37	40	43
5'6"	-	22	24	26	28	30	32	34	35	40	42
5'7"	-	15	20	22	24	26	28	30	32	34	37
5'8"	-	-	18	20	22	24	26	28	30	32	34
5'9"	-	-	-	18	20	22	24	26	28	30	32
5'10"	-	-	-	-	18	20	22	24	26	28	30

TABLE 4

For Average Females Who Exercise 5 Times Per Week

(Including Aerobics and Resistance Training)

	WEIGHT										
HEIGHT	100	110	120	130	140	150	160	170	180	190	200
5'	18	24	26	28	30	32	34	-	-	-	-
5'1"	16	22	24	26	28	30	32	-	-	-	-
5'2"	15	22	24	26	26	28	30	-	-	-	-
5'3"	15	19	20	22	24	27	29	31	33	35	37
5'4"	15	17	21	23	25	26	28	30	32	34	36
5'5"	-	16	19	22	24	26	28	30	32	34	35
5'6"	-	-	18	20	22	24	26	28	30	32	34
5'7"	-	-	16	18	21	24	26	28	30	32	33
5'8"	-	-	14	17	20	23	25	27	29	30	32
5'9"	-	-	-	15	18	20	22	24	26	28	30
5'10"	-	-	-	15	18	20	22	24	26	28	29

Planning Meals

Now that you have computed your daily protein requirement (and other nutritional needs) let's look at how you can use your DPR to estimate the amount you should eat at each meal. Here are some suggestions on how to distribute your protein intake throughout the day. Remember, these are just suggestions!

76 grams of protein daily

Breakfast	14 grams
Lunch	20 grams
Snack	7 grams
Dinner	35 grams

81 grams of protein daily

Breakfast	14 grams
Lunch	25 grams
Snack	7 grams
Dinner	35 grams

83 grams of protein daily

Breakfast	14 grams
Snack	7 grams
Lunch	20 grams
Snack	7 grams
Dinner	35 grams

88 grams of protein daily

Breakfast	14 grams
Snack	7 grams
Lunch	25 grams
Snack	7 grams
Dinner	35 grams

96 grams of protein daily

Breakfast	14 grams
Lunch	35 grams
Snack	7 grams
Dinner	40 grams

103 grams of protein daily

Breakfast	14 grams
Snack	7 grams
Lunch	35 grams
Snack	7 grams
Dinner	40 grams

113 grams of protein daily

Breakfast	17 grams
Snack	7 grams
Lunch	35 grams
Snack	14 grams
Dinner	40 grams

120 grams of protein daily

Breakfast	17 grams
Snack	14 grams
Lunch	35 grams
Snack	14 grams
Dinner	40 grams

128 grams of protein daily

Breakfast	17 grams
Snack	7 grams
Lunch	45 grams
Snack	14 grams
Dinner	45 grams

135 grams of protein daily

Breakfast	17 grams
Snack	14 grams
Lunch	45 grams
Snack	14 grams
Dinner	45 grams

146 grams of protein daily

Breakfast	35 grams
Snack	7 grams
Lunch	45 grams
Snack	14 grams
Dinner	45 grams

153 grams of protein daily

Breakfast	35 grams
Snack	14 grams
Lunch	45 grams
Snack	14 grams
Dinner	45 grams

158 grams of protein daily

Breakfast	35 grams
Snack	14 grams
Lunch	45 grams
Snack	14 grams
Dinner	50 grams

So what is a meal that contains 14 grams of protein and a balance of other macronutrients? A meal with 45 grams of protein? With a little experience, you'll be able to tell how much protein and other nutrients are in a typical meal. Here are a few examples. Use them to develop a sense of what a good meal contains.

BREAKFAST
Approximately 14 grams of protein

Example 1

A nutrition bar (a Balance bar for example)

22 gm carbohydrates, 15 gm protein, 6 gm fat

190 calories

Example 2
Scrambled eggs (1 whole, 2 whites)
1 slice whole wheat toast
1 peach
23 gm carbohydrates, 14 gm protein, 6 gm fat
200 calories

Example 3
1/2 bagel
1/2 oz cream cheese
1 1/2 oz sliced turkey
1/2 orange
23 gm carbohydrates, 15 gm protein, 8 gm fat
224 calories

Approximately 35 grams of protein

Example 1
6-egg omelet (2 whole eggs, 4 whites)
1 3/4 cups cooked oatmeal
1/2 cup low-fat milk
52 gm. carbohydrates, 39 gm protein, 18 gm fat
526 calories

Example 2
6-egg omelet (2 whole eggs, 4 whites)
2 slices whole wheat toast
1 tbsp peanut butter
1 small low-glycemic fruit (see below)
43 gm carbohydrates, 31 gm protein, 15 gm fat
431 calories

Example 3

1 cup low-fat cottage cheese

1/2 bagel

1/4 of a medium avocado

1/2 small low-glycemic fruit

41 gm carbohydrates, 30 gm protein, 12 gm fat

392 calories

LUNCH
Approximately 20 grams of protein

Example 1

3/4 cup low-fat cottage cheese

1 piece of low-glycemic fruit

1 tbsp almonds

29 gm carbohydrates, 21 gm protein, 11 gm fat

299 calories

Example 2

2.5 oz sliced turkey or chicken breast

lettuce and tomato

1/2 pita pocket

1/2 tbsp mayonnaise

1/2 piece low-glycemic fruit

26 gm carbohydrates, 19 gm protein, 9 gm fat

259 calories

Example 3

3 oz water-packed tuna

lettuce and tomato

1 slice bread

1/2 tbsp mayonnaise

1 small low-glycemic fruit

28 gm carbohydrates, 22 gm protein, 10 gm fat

290 calories

Approximately 35 grams of protein

Example 1

4.5 oz sliced turkey or chicken breast

lettuce and tomato

2 slices bread

2 tsp mayonnaise

1 piece low-glycemic fruit

45 gm carbohydrates, 34 gm protein, 16 gm fat

460 calories

Example 2

4.5 oz water-packed tuna salad

(pickles, celery, onions, and 1 tbsp mayonnaise)

lettuce and tomato

1 pita pocket

1 small low-glycemic fruit

47 gm carbohydrates, 34 gm protein, 16 gm fat

468 calories

Example 3

5 oz chicken, turkey, tuna, or 1 cup low-fat cottage cheese

1 large salad with 2 tbsp dressing

1 slice whole wheat bread

1 large low-glycemic fruit

47 gm carbohydrates, 36 gm protein, 17 gm fat, 485 calories

Approximately 45 grams of protein

Example 1

6.5 oz water-packed tuna

1 cup cooked pasta with 1 tbsp olive oil

1 cup cooked low-glycemic vegetables (see below)

65 gm carbohydrates, 49 gm protein, 22 gm fat

654 calories

Example 2

6 oz skinned chicken or turkey breast

2 slices whole wheat bread

lettuce, tomato, and cucumber slices

1 tbsp mayonnaise

1 large low-glycemic fruit

59 gm carbohydrates, 44 gm protein, 21 gm fat

601 calories

DINNER
Approximately 35 grams of protein

Example 1

4 oz baked or broiled halibut

1/2 cup cooked pasta

1 1/2 cups cooked low-glycemic vegetables

1 large dinner salad with 2 tbsp dressing

45 gm carbohydrates, 34 gm protein, 15 gm fat, 451 calories
Example 2

4.5 oz baked or broiled chicken breast

1/2 baked potato

1 cup cooked low-glycemic vegetables

1 large dinner salad with 2 tbsp dressing

47 gm carbohydrates, 36 gm protein, 16 gm fat

476 calories

Example 3

4.5 oz lean ground turkey

3/4 cup cooked pasta with 1/2 cup marinara sauce

1/2 cup cooked low-glycemic vegetables

48 gm carbohydrates, 36 gm protein, 17 gm fat

489 calories

Example 4

3 oz lean pork loin

1 1/2 cups broccoli

1 cup zucchini

1/4 cup peas

1/2 red or green bell pepper

1/2 cup cooked rice

1 tsp olive or canola oil (to stir-fry ingredients)

46 gm carbohydrates, 35 gm protein, 17 gm fat

477 calories

Approximately 40 grams of protein

Example 1

5 oz baked or broiled halibut

1/2 baked potato

2 cups cooked low-glycemic vegetables

1 large dinner salad with 1 tbsp dressing

57 gm carbohydrates, 43 gm protein, 19 gm fat

571 calories

Example 2

5 oz baked or broiled skinless chicken breast

1/2 cup cooked rice

2 cups cooked low-glycemic vegetables

1 large dinner salad with 2 tbsp dressing

52 gm carbohydrates, 39 gm protein, 17 gm fat

517 calories

Example 3

5 oz lean ground turkey

3/4 cup cooked pasta with 1/2 cup marinara sauce

1 cup cooked low-glycemic vegetables

53 gm carbohydrates, 40 gm protein, 18 gm fat

534 calories

Example 4

3.5 oz lean pork loin

1 1/2 cups broccoli

1 1/2 cups zucchini

1/2 cup peas

1/2 of a red or green bell pepper

1/2 cup cooked rice

1 tsp olive or canola oil (to stir-fry ingredients)

53 gm carbohydrates, 41 gm protein, 19 gm fat

547 calories

Approximately 45 grams of protein

Example 1

5.5 oz baked or broiled halibut

1 1/4 cups cooked low-glycemic vegetables

1 cup cooked pasta

1 large dinner salad with 1 tbsp dressing

63 gm carbohydrates, 46 gm protein, 22 gm fat

634 calories

Example 2

6 oz skinned chicken or turkey breast

3/4 cup cooked rice

1 1/2 cups cooked low-glycemic vegetables

1 large dinner salad with 1 tbsp dressing

58 gm carbohydrates, 45 gm protein, 22 gm fat

610 calories

SNACKS

Example 1

1 nutrition bar

A typical nutrition bar, like a Balance bar, is a good snack thirty minutes before a workout, between meals, or thirty minutes before bed. A Balance bar breaks down as follows (for other brands, read the label):

19 gm carbohydrates, 14 gm protein, 6 gm fat

Example 2

1 slice whole wheat bread

1 tsp mayonnaise

1 oz turkey

13 gm carbohydrates, 10 gm protein, 5 gm fat

Example 3

1/2 cup low-fat cottage cheese

1 cup diced melon or diced pineapple

22 gm carbohydrates, 14 gm protein, 5 gm fat

LOW-GLYCEMIC MEALS

Not all carbohydrates are equal in terms of the rate at which our body breaks down and absorbs them. The slower the rate of carbohydrate digestion, the better. Foods that are digested quickly, and make our blood sugar rise rapidly, have what is called a high-glycemic index. Those that are absorbed more slowly have a low-glycemic index, and those in the middle a moderate-glycemic index. Foods with the highest index include things like white bread, most cereals, corn, honey, and simple sugar. Moderate-glycemic foods include most pastas, whole-grain breads, rice, oatmeal, and peas. The following is a list of low-glycemic carbohydrates.

Low-Glycemic Grains

Barley
Oatmeal (the slow-cooking variety)
Sourdough
Whole-grain Rye Bread

Other Low-Glycemic Foods

Peanuts
Skim milk
Yogurt

Low-Glycemic Vegetables

Artichokes	Cucumbers	Lima Beans
Asparagus	Eggplant	Soybeans
Broccoli	Garbanzo Beans	Spinach
Brussels Sprouts	Green Beans	Tomatoes
Cabbage	Kidney Beans	Zucchini
Cauliflower	Lentils	
Celery	Lettuce	

Low-Glycemic Fruits

Apples	Grapefruit	Pears
Cherries	Oranges	Plums
Grapes	Peaches	Strawberries

Balanced Low-Glycemic Meals

If you want to really maximize your weight loss, you might try eating a diet of low-glycemic foods for a while. Here are six sample meals:

Example 1

One 6 oz can water-packed tuna

1/4 cup celery

1 oz pickle relish

2 tbsp reduced-fat mayo

Mix above ingredients and serve with:

2 cups shredded lettuce

2 Rykrisp crackers

1 medium apple

56 gm carbohydrates, 43 gm protein, 15 gm fat

540 calories

Example 2

4 oz water-packed tuna

1 medium tangerine

1 medium kiwi

2 Rykrisp crackers

3 cups romaine lettuce with 2 tbsp oil and vinegar dressing

49 gm carbohydrates, 37 gm protein, 8 gm fat

426 calories

Example 3

1 cup low-fat cottage cheese

2 cups shredded lettuce

1 cup sprouts

1 large sliced apple

1 tbsp granola, sprinkled on top

41 gm carbohydrates, 32 gm protein, 9 gm fat, 374 calories

Example 4

3 1/2 oz chicken or lean beef

1 cup broccoli

1/2 cup snow peas

1 medium red or green bell pepper

1 sliced green onion

1/2 cup bean sprouts

1 tsp extra virgin olive oil (to stir-fry ingredients)

1 medium orange

53 gm carbohydrates, 40 gm protein, 13 gm fat

489 calories

Example 5

4 oz extra lean ground beef

1 cup steamed broccoli

1/2 cup steamed cauliflower

1 fresh steamed artichoke

Dip made of 1 tsp Dijon mustard and 1 tbsp reduced-fat mayo

1 medium orange

59 gm carbohydrates, 46 gm protein, 18 gm fat

580 calories

Example 6

1 cup low-fat cottage cheese

1 steamed zucchini

1/2 sliced cucumber

1/2 large tomato broiled with 1 tbsp Parmesan cheese and garlic

1 medium orange

56 gm carbohydrates, 43 gm protein, 9 gm fat

477 calories

A Note to Athletes

Most of you who are reading this book—if you are true to the demographics of contemporary America—have not yet begun the journey to health. But there are some of you who may already be on the road. For those who are dedicated exercisers and athletes, the balanced nutritional approach I have described may need to be modified. If you are already fit, it's advisable to move up one level in your daily protein requirement (DPR), to make sure you are getting the nutrients you need to maintain a stable weight and body fat percentage. Some athletes require more protein in their diets than 30 percent, but few require less. A balanced diet will help you recover more quickly from strenuous workouts and competitions, lower your injury rate, and improve your energy level. This is particularly true for men and women who are endurance athletes.

If you are a long-distance runner, cyclist, or swimmer, a bi- or triathlete, the benefits of a long-term, balanced diet will show up in markedly improved performance. Many world-class endurance athletes, who are now eating a balanced diet, are able to maintain a higher level of exertion for a longer period of time. Preliminary studies at three major universities show that a balanced diet can give endurance athletes the ability to access up to 80 percent of their energy needs from stored fat. Athletes on a high-carbohydrate diet were able to access only about 40 percent of their energy from stored fat. As we know, the liver can store only so much glycogen. The athlete who depends less on stored glycogen and more on stored fat will have much better endurance.

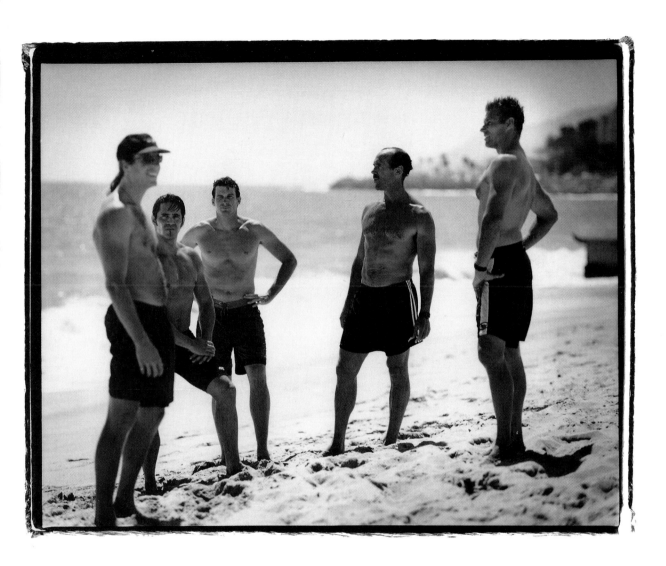

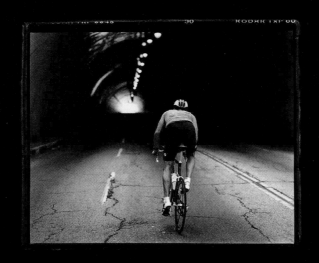

I advised a lot of people at Gold's Gym and eventually built a good reputation in the local health and fitness community. One day in November 1981, a prominent entertainment attorney approached me. He had just broken up with his girlfriend and was deeply depressed. He wanted to make some fundamental changes in his life and offered me twenty-five dollars an hour to help him get in shape. It seemed like an enormous fee. I accepted. With my first paying customer, I had embarked on a new career—although I didn't know it. The term "personal trainer" wasn't in widespread use yet. The attorney turned out to be an ideal client. He took several weeks off and did little else but train. In a month and a half, he seemed transformed. He returned to work, pulled up his shirt, and showed off his abs to the other attorneys. He had new found energy. He wasn't depressed. My client roster quickly filled up with his colleagues. Some just wanted to lose a few pounds, but others wanted to look like Tarzan. I got results for all of them.

EXERCISE
ENHANCES BODY AND SOUL

Exercise, like diet, has significance for our whole being. For millennia, yoga, sacred and ritual dance, tribal rites of passage, and other forms of movement have celebrated the body's relation to the soul. When seen from the perspective of history, exercise has not been performed in clinical detachment—movement has been closely related to worship. Practitioners of yoga know that exercise quiets the mind, refreshes the body, and frees the spirit. Moshe Feldenkrais, among others, has taught us that every inner experience is also a bodily experience. The ancient Chinese meditative exercise T'ai Chi Ch'uan affirms the intimate relationship of body and mind. The most common metaphor for the spiritual life in Christianity is the journey—a physical process that involves walking, climbing, and moving around obstacles. Madonna's remark that exercise is like church reveals a deep understanding of its significance. The full benefits of exercise cannot be measured in strictly clinical terms. Its effects extend to the soul.

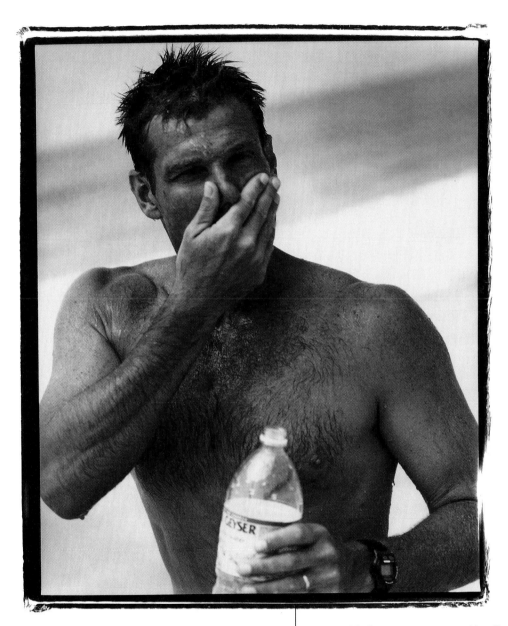

exercise the soul

Mind and body are not seperate entities. Every inner experience is also a bodily experience, and every bodily experience affects the soul.

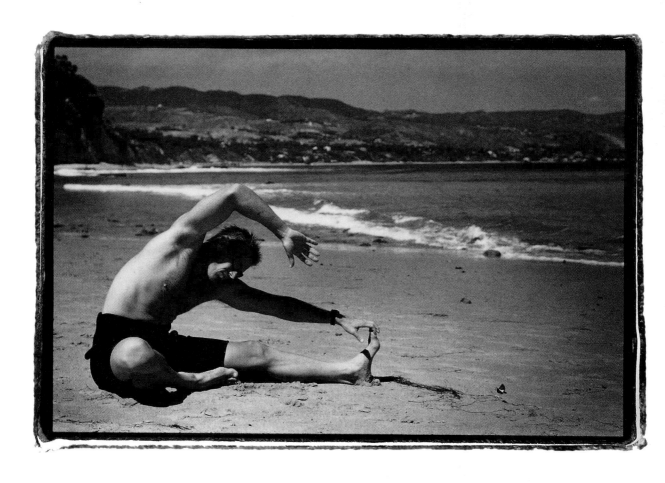

a calling

The journey toward health is a
response to an inner voice.

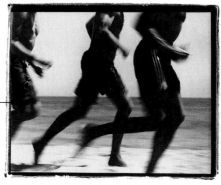

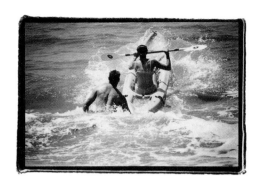

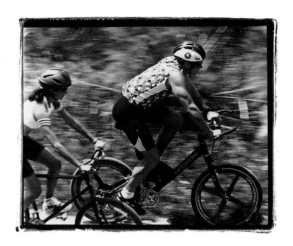

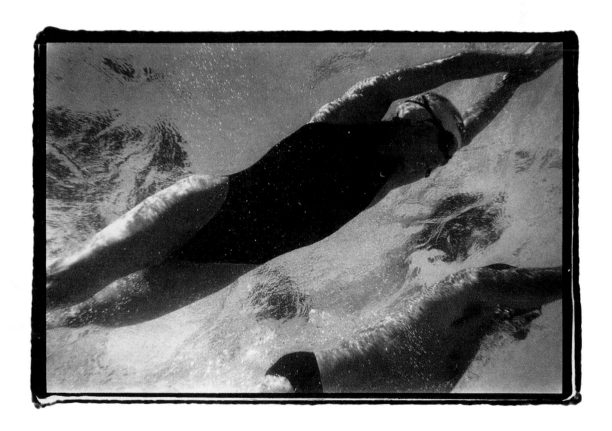

Monks and religious contemplatives traditionally refer to their spiritual journey as a "vocation," from the Latin word meaning "to call." In other words, the spiritual journey is a response to an inner voice, a calling. And so it is with the journey toward health. A physical regimen that endures over time is the inevitable response to a powerful voice from within. After a time, most of my clients develop a zeal for exercise that is so powerful it cannot be ignored. They become ardent advocates for a vigorous, athletic lifestyle. The psychological and spiritual benefits they gain from exercise provide them with the discipline to keep on going. Others—the unbelievers—who exercise out of a sense of guilt, vanity, or the desire to achieve short-term goals, inevitably fail. Without an inner conviction the discipline necessary to continue flags. But believers never tire of the journey because they know and have experienced the life-giving benefits of exercise.

"People who exercise understand the rational, scientific basis of its benefits, but they also know and experience its virtues in a way that transcends reason."

Passion—another religious term—has meaning for those who live a physically active life, too. People who exercise understand the rational, scientific basis of its benefits, but they also know and experience its virtues in a way that transcends reason. Madonna and I have pursued health through exercise so long and enjoyed its benefits so profoundly that we have a developed a passion for it. When you are passionate about what you do, success is assured. When you try to sustain a fitness program through sheer force of will, you neither enjoy the journey nor have the

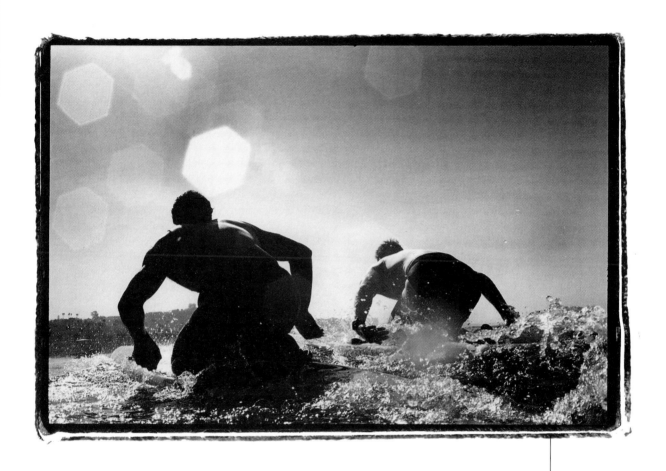

a passion

With passion, success is assured;

without it, you will fail.

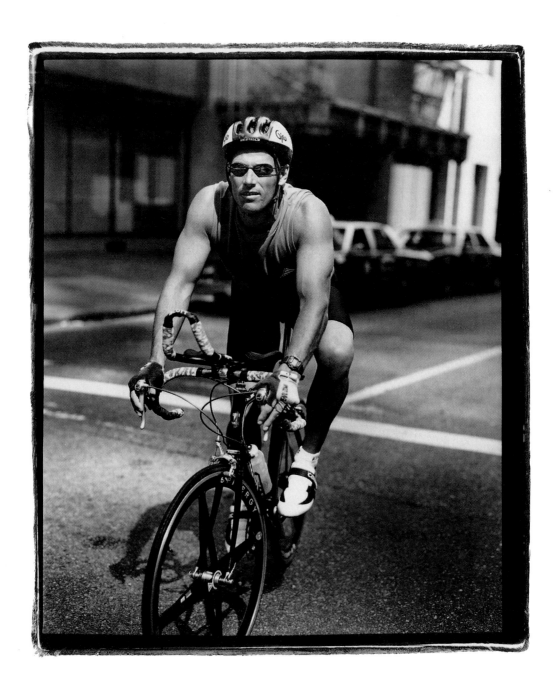

power to sustain it. Steely determination is no substitute for love. Love produces another kind of commitment—the kind you can keep.

"In spite of all the rhetoric about the need to live an active, healthy lifestyle, few Americans have heeded the call."

In 1995 the American College of Sports Medicine estimated that as many as 250,000 Americans die prematurely every year because of their sedentary habits. To put this in perspective, five times as many people succumb annually to the effects of their inactive lifestyles than are killed in automobile accidents. The old biblical statement that "many are called but few are chosen" applies equally to health and religion. According to the Centers for Disease Control almost 60 percent of Americans are physically inactive and less than 10 percent exercise intensively. In spite of all the rhetoric about the need to live an active, healthy lifestyle, few Americans have heeded the call. Most have chosen a life of destructive self-indulgence. But why? The benefits of exercise are not insignificant. A California Department of Health study estimated that an active lifestyle could add eleven years to the life of an average man and seven to a woman. As a past president of the American College of Sports Medicine has said, "The active life is not one of denial and deprivation, nor is it one of pain and hurt. It is a joyful experience, an affirmation of what we can be physically, mentally, socially, and spiritually."

"Like diet, exercise will make significant changes to your body's chemistry and physiological systems."

My analysis of the health literature suggests that even moderate exercise, if done consistently, will help immunize you to some degree against heart disease, adult-onset diabetes, hypertension, some kinds of cancer, osteoporosis, and the more debilitating symptoms of aging. Like diet, exercise will make significant changes to your body's chemistry and physiological systems. However, most conventional physicians will admit that regular exercise helps control obesity, blood pressure, and cholesterol levels—and little else. Medicine is a very conservative discipline and highly resistant to change. Grudgingly, however, the medical community is admitting to an ever-increasing list of significant benefits. Scientists who study the effects of exercise on the body—the people on the cutting edge of research—are expanding the list all the time. Here are the main physical and psychological benefits of exercise that have emerged in studies over the past several years.

A healthier heart.

Regular exercise will make your heart more efficient, stronger, and better able to supply your body with blood. When you are fit, your heart is able to utilize oxygen more effectively and beat at a lower rate. Your heart is a muscle, and when that muscle is conditioned it doesn't have to work as hard. Fit people have lower resting and exercise heart rates than unfit people. Fit people also have what is called a higher stroke volume—their hearts pump more blood with each beat. The blood supply to the heart muscle itself is also improved when you are fit. Even if you are prone to clogged coronary arteries, exercise may enlarge and strengthen them and make you less susceptible to arteriosclerosis.

Reduced hypertension.

Unfit people are much more likely to have high blood pressure and the many health risks associated with it. People with high blood pressure are at four times the risk of developing congestive heart failure than others. If you exercise regularly, you will reduce the chances of developing hypertension by at least one-third. Even if you do suffer from high blood pressure, if you exercise you will reduce your risk of serious consequences by one-half. One of the significant risks of hypertension is a stroke. Regular moderate exercise for people with high blood pressure will substantially reduce the risk of a stroke. In fact, there is an inverse relationship between strokes and activity—the more you exercise, the less the risk.

Improved circulation.

In addition to the heart itself, blood must flow efficiently through your vascular system, the network of veins and arteries that deliver life-giving fluid to every cell in your body. If you get regular aerobic exercise, you can increase your blood volume by as much as 15 percent. Increased volume reduces the load on your heart, delivers more blood to your muscles, and reduces blood pressure during exercise. Exercise also improves the elasticity of blood vessels and makes them less vulnerable to damage. Regular exercise can also help to prevent blood clots, a factor that becomes increasingly important as we age.

Better fat metabolism.

Exercise is the best way to get your body to burn fat for energy. If you diet you'll likely lose muscle tissue, which in the long run is highly counterproductive. Regular exercise requires your body to burn more calories and trains it to mobilize and metabolize fat. Additionally, exercise builds muscle which raises your basal metabolism, making your body an ever more efficient fat burner. Regular exercise also stimulates the body to produce a good kind of cholesterol, called HDL (high-density lipoprotein). HDL's function in the body is to scour fatty deposits, the so-called bad cholesterol (LDL, or low-density lipoprotein), from your arteries and transport it to your liver for disposal. Finally, regular physical activity will reduce the amount of fatty acids (triglycerides) circulating in your blood.

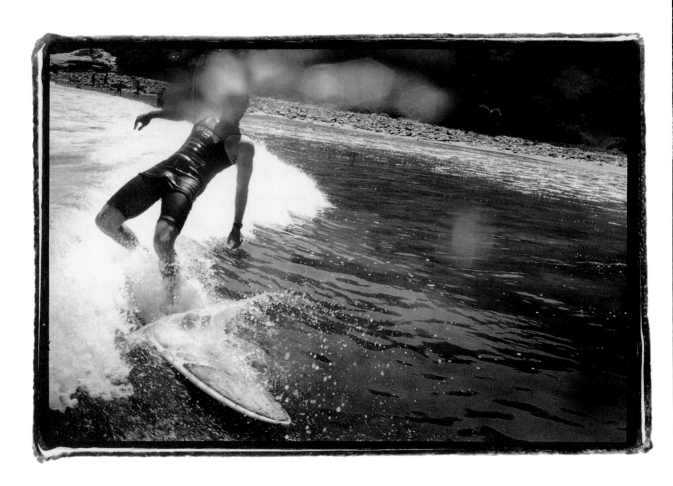

Resistance to adult-onset diabetes.

When you exercise regularly your body becomes more sensitive to insulin and more tolerant of blood glucose levels. When you have too much fat circulating in your blood system, insulin cannot transport glucose to your muscles very efficiently. Adult-onset (type II) diabetes has become a major problem for aging baby boomers and the elderly, yet it is completely preventable for most people and rare among those who are fit. Type II diabetes is a disease closely related to lifestyle and personal choice. The price to pay for a self-indulgent, sedentary lifestyle may be an old age of chronic illness. Active adults have a 42 percent lower risk of developing type II diabetes.

An improved skeletal system.

Exercise in general, and resistance training in particular, will improve your body's utilization of calcium. People who lift weights, even moderate weights, have thicker, stronger bones. Osteoporosis, the loss of bone minerals common in many postmenopausal women, is accelerated by a lack of exercise. Women who are fit—and stay fit for life—are unlikely candidates for later problems with osteoporosis. The effects of arthritis are also diminished through exercise. People who exercise are less likely to develop arthritis, and those who do can substantially relieve their symptoms by keeping active. The chronic back and spine problems that beset so many sedentary people can be minimized and often reversed through exercise.

An improved immune system.

Scientists are still arguing this one out, but it seems that a healthy lifestyle does help prevent certain types of cancer. For example, exercise

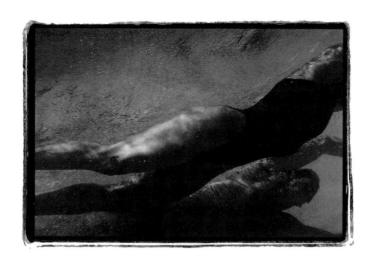

may reduce the chance of breast and uterine cancer in women and prostate cancer in men. There seems to be a link between low body fat and resistance to some kinds of cancer. Regular exercise definitely enhances the operation of the immune system; however, excessive exercise is just another form of stress and can actually suppress the immune system. If you're having fun being fit, it is unlikely that you will exercise to excess. When you are relaxed in body and mind, your immune system has a chance to operate at maximum effectiveness.

An improved sense of well-being.

Ask anyone who exercises regularly and they will tell you that the world just doesn't seem right when they miss a day of working out. Madonna's statement in chapter one that she "just wouldn't feel right" if she didn't exercise is completely consistent with the experience of others on the journey of fitness. Exercise is like a drug—the world's best antidepressant! In fact, if it were a drug it would, as one researcher has put it, "be hailed as a modern miracle." Studies have shown that regular exercise reduces anxiety levels, decreases feelings of depression, and improves self-esteem.

ALWAYS SEEK
BALANCE

Many athletes, particularly runners, speak of exercise as a *Positive Addiction*—the name of a book written more than two decades ago by Dr. William Glasser. Glasser argued convincingly that runners, as well as people who practice yoga and other contemplative disciplines, develop positive addictions that enable them to be stronger, more imaginative, and more creative. I know many people who consider themselves to be addicted to physical activity. An addiction to fitness, however, is life-giving in distinction to the many life-*threatening* habits that afflict our society.

So how do we attain all of these wonderful benefits? Through a balanced exercise program that achieves both aerobic and muscular fitness. Aerobic exercise, a term coined in 1967 by Dr. Kenneth Cooper, is usually defined as exercise below the level at which your body is able to efficiently oxidize a byproduct of muscular exertion called lactic acid. In practical terms, this means exercise below the threshold of discomfort. If you are jogging, for example, at a level at which you can continue indefinitely, or at a level at which you can talk without too much effort, you are exercising aerobically. If you are running uphill, out of breath and uncomfortable, you have probably crossed the threshold into what is called anaerobic exercise. When you exercise aerobically, your body burns mostly fats and some carbohydrates. When you cross the threshold into anaerobic exercise, you burn mostly carbohydrates and not much fat. Aerobic fitness will improve your cardiovascular system, and hence your physical endurance.

> "The foundation of any exercise program is a regular regimen of aerobic activity."

Muscular fitness is the result of exercise that increases muscle mass. Muscular fitness is achieved through exercises that involve resistance and is sometimes called "resistance training." Weight training is the most common method of achieving muscular fitness. The goal of this type of exercise is to increase muscular endurance, strength, flexibility, agility, coordination, and balance. The benefits of muscular fitness include raising your basal metabolism (so you burn more fat), strengthening your skeletal system, increasing your athleticism, and mitigating the effects of age.

The foundation of any exercise program is a regular regimen of aerobic activity. People who are unfit and begin a program of aerobic exercise often find their lives transformed. They lose weight and look better; they have more energy; and they become more productive. Running, speed walking, cycling, rowing, paddling, in-line skating, and cross-country skiing are all great fun and, at the same time, excellent ways to achieve aerobic fitness. Each of these activities will improve your heart and lungs and strengthen large muscle groups. All of these experiences can also have the potential to be social and aesthetic experiences, by getting you outside with friends in beautiful natural settings.

a balanced regimen

Every exercise program should include exercises that achieve both muscular and aerobic fitness.

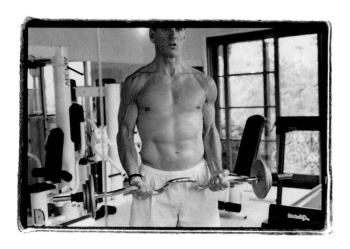

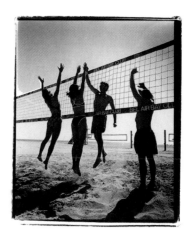

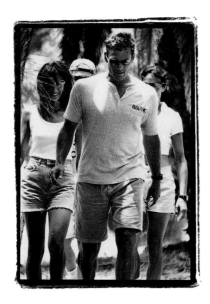

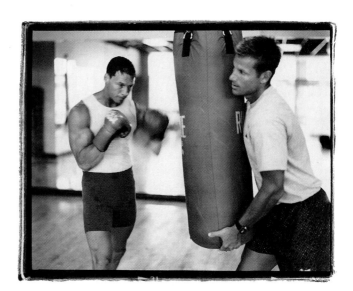

125

"Whatever exercise or combination of exercises you choose, the key to achieving good results is learning to control the level of intensity."

There are many wonderful aerobic exercises that you can do. What you choose will depend to some degree on where you live. I live near the beach, so my favorite workout is to run a few miles in the soft sand by the water's edge, return and get my paddle board, and do another mile or so on the water. With this combination I work my legs intensively for a while and then my upper body. When I'm done, I feel exhilarated. I often do this routine with friends and make my workout a social occasion. I much prefer outdoor exercise to aerobic work in a gym. In California this is possible year round. Weather permitting, wherever you live, outdoor exercise that involves propelling yourself by means of your own energy is always the most rewarding. Self-propelling exercises include running, cycling, swimming, hiking, cross-country skiing, paddleboarding, kayaking, rowing, and outrigger canoeing—anything that gets you from point "A" to point "B" under your own power and with an elevated heart rate. If the weather keeps you inside, you can use a VersaCimber, StairMaster, Lifecycle or treadmill— these will give you a good workout, but won't be as much fun as outdoor activities. If you're stuck inside, do your aerobic work with a friend—the time will go by much more quickly.

"Within the training zone, the benefits you experience will vary according to intensity."

Whatever exercise or combination of exercises you choose, the key to achieving good results is learning to control the level of intensity. There are many ways to measure intensity, but for the layperson the most practical is to monitor your heart rate. I often use a heart-rate monitor, an item that can be purchased inexpensively from most any sporting goods store. The idea is to monitor your heart rate to determine when you have entered what is called the "training zone." Exercise that is too low in intensity will not give you good results, and neither will exercise that is too strenuous. Within the training zone, the benefits you will experience vary according to intensity. At the low end of the zone, your body's ability to metabolize fat is optimized; at the upper end the benefits are mostly cardiovascular. If you vary your activity level within the aerobic, or training zone, occasionally pushing the upper limit, you will gradually raise your level of cardiovascular fitness. If you don't push the upper limit of your training zone once in while, you will still enjoy many benefits but you won't improve or raise your aerobic threshold. Periodically pushing the upper limit of your training zone is called "interval training." Interval training should comprise about 15 to 20 percent of your aerobic workout.

The American College of Sports Medicine has developed a handy little acronym to remember the basic elements of a good aerobic fitness program: FIT. FIT stands for *Frequency, Intensity* and *Time*. Sometimes a fourth "T" is added to stand for *Type*.

Frequency.

A good aerobic program should include a minimum of three days of exercise per week, and a maximum of five. If you are a beginner and out of shape, a brisk walk three times a week will get you on the road to health. If

"The purpose of interval training is to overload your system by gradually increasing the duration and intensity of your workout."

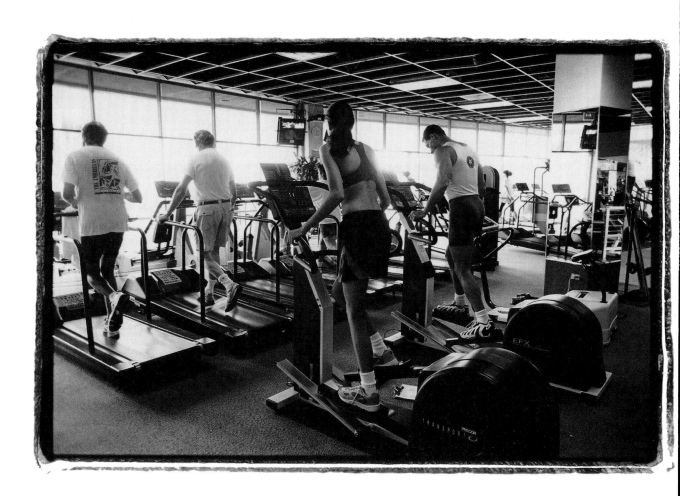

you are a hard-core runner, more than five days a week of training will gain you little additional benefit and put you at risk for injury.

Intensity.

Whatever form of exercise you choose, it should raise your heart rate into the training zone of 70 to 85 percent of your maximum.

Time.

If you are just starting a program, you should aim for a minimum of fifteen minutes in the training zone. If you are already aerobically fit, the American College of Sports Medicine recommends that you limit your time in the zone to an hour. Unless you're training for an endurance race, an hour is plenty of time in the training zone.

Type.

The type of exercise you do must be truly aerobic, which means an activity that is continuous and that uses large muscle groups. This rules out golf, billiards, and croquet, but includes many other fun activities (don't give up your nonaerobic sports, just add something more strenuous).

So how do you monitor your heart rate and figure out when you're in the training zone? A wristwatch and a pulse is all the equipment you need. If you don't have a pulse, then you're reading this book too late! The easiest place to feel your pulse is at your carotid artery, right next to your windpipe. Place two fingers lightly on your neck adjacent to your windpipe and just under your chin; count the beats for ten seconds, and multiply by six. Practice until you get the hang of it. Next, you need to determine what your theoretical maximum heart rate is.

This is easy. Write the number 220 on a piece of paper and under it, your age. Subtract. The resulting number is your maximum heart rate. Now calculate your training zone. To do this, multiply your maximum heart rate by 70 percent and 85 percent and round off the numbers. Here's how it would work for a forty-year-old.

ESTABLISHING THE TRAINING ZONE FOR A FORTY-YEAR-OLD

1. CALCULATE YOUR MAXIMUM HEART RATE:

220 (reference number)

-40 (your age)

180 (your maximum heart rate)

2. CALCULATE YOUR TRAINING ZONE:

180 (your maximum heart rate) x 70% (lower aerobic limit) = 126

180 (your maximum heart rate) x 85% (upper aerobic limit = 153

3. WRITE DOWN YOUR TRAINING ZONE:

Your training zone is between 126 and 153.

A heart-rate monitor is a really good way to keep in the training zone, because it gives you continuous feedback. A typical sports-type heart-rate monitor is a two-piece affair that includes a strap with a sensor/transmitter attached to it that goes around your chest and a receiving unit that looks like a digital wristwatch. Most monitors have a built-in alarm that allows you to set your upper and lower aerobic heart rates. If you drop below or rise above your training zone, an alarm beeps.

fitness is progressive

Push yourself, but remember that fitness is a long-term commitment.

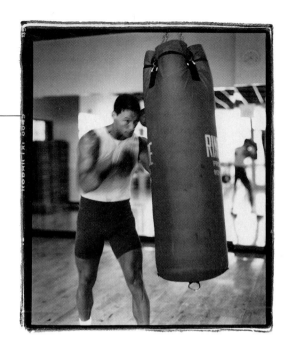

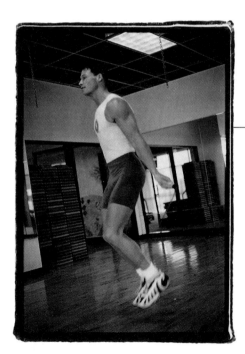

it takes a lifetime

If you train too hard, too fast, you'll probably burn out.

If you drop dead, it lets out a continuous tone. Just kidding. Most units are waterproof, so you can take them swimming or paddleboarding, too.

"The purpose of interval training is to overload your system by gradually increasing the duration and intensity of your workout."

Okay, so you've done the calculations and established your personal training zone. What next? If you're a beginner, I recommend you start off by doing fifteen to twenty minutes of aerobic exercise a day, three days a week, always keeping your heart rate in the training zone. As your fitness improves, increase the length of your workout and add days. If you're particularly fit, five or even six days a week of aerobic workouts (no more

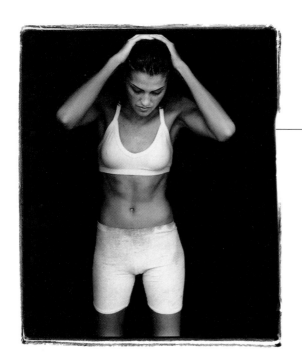

discomfort not pain

Discomfort is normal, but pain is not.
Persistent pain is a sign that something's wrong.

than an hour per day) is optimum. However many days you exercise, at least 15 percent of your workout should be interval training. You can do your interval training either on a daily basis or on a weekly basis. Some people like to set aside a portion of each daily workout as interval training while others prefer to do their interval training one or two days a week. Either way, just make sure the total time adds up to approximately 15 percent of your total aerobic workout time.

"Interval training is a kind of controlled discomfort, in which you take your body to the limit and push on to a higher level."

So how do you do interval training? It's easy. Let's say you've chosen running as your aerobic exercise. If you run for thirty minutes, set aside about five minutes to elevate your heart rate up to the top of your training zone. To do this, simply speed up your pace until your heart rate reaches 85 percent of its maximum (this is where a heart-rate monitor is really handy) and keep it there for one minute. After the minute is up, slow down (don't stop!) for thirty seconds and let your heart rate go back down. Then repeat the cycle—one minute on and thirty seconds off—until you've kept your pulse at 85 percent of your maximum for a total of five minutes. Most any aerobic activity lends itself to this kind of on-off cycle.

"While discomfort is a normal byproduct of interval training, pain is not."

The purpose of interval training is to overload your system by gradually increasing the duration and intensity of your workout. When you overload your body's systems for short periods of time, it changes to accommodate for future demands. Your circulation improves and becomes more efficient at supplying your muscles with energy; protein is mobilized to build new muscle tissue; and your nervous system learns to recruit more muscle fibers with greater effectiveness. At first, interval training will seem daunting. It will make you uncomfortable, and many people are afraid of discomfort. But as your fitness improves, you will grow in confidence, too, and learn to deal with it. Interval training is a kind of controlled discomfort, in which you take your body to the limit and push on to a higher level. After a while the discomfort becomes its own reward as you learn to associate it with growth and progress. Remember, you are in control of your workout, and you can dial the intensity up or down at any time you want. Just keep in mind that fitness is progressive. Push yourself, but always remember that aerobic health is a long-term commitment. You don't have to achieve Olympic levels of fitness overnight—or ever. You have a lifetime to get and remain fit. Don't rush things. It takes years of training to reach the highest levels of fitness. If you train too hard, too fast, you'll probably burn out. Interval training will help you make progress in your aerobic fitness program, but it will do so gradually. Enjoy and celebrate each milestone on the journey of fitness.

"Everyone who engages in a program of regular aerobic exercise and interval training will achieve significant health gains."

While discomfort is a normal byproduct of interval training, pain is not. The "no pain, no gain" slogan is not really true. It shouldn't hurt. Persistent or sharp pain is a sign that something's wrong. If you experience real pain, as distinguished from discomfort, back off or stop what you are doing. When you work out, your body produces substances called endorphins. Endorphins act like morphine, a potent analgesic drug. Endorphins make you feel exhilarated and are responsible for the phenomenon known as "runner's high." Any physical distress that is powerful enough to override these natural painkillers during exercise is something you must pay attention to.

Everyone who engages in a program of regular aerobic exercise and interval training will achieve significant health gains. But there are some factors you should keep in mind, so that the goals you set for yourself are realistic. Remember, the goal is health, not the achievement of certain statistical objectives. Go easy on yourself. If you set unrealistic standards you'll be disappointed. The journey itself is the reward. There are some things you can't change, and it doesn't make any sense to try. Here are the factors that will influence the upper limits of what you can achieve.

renew yourself

The combination of strength and aerobic training can revitalize you in surprising and powerful ways.

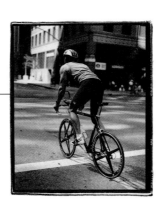

Heredity.

It has been said that the best way to become a world-class athlete is to choose your parents wisely. Some people are genetically endowed for long-distance or endurance events, and others are well suited to athletic feats that require explosive power. Studies of aerobic capacity have concluded that 25 to 50 percent of our ability is inherited—the other 50 to 75 percent is the result of diet and training. If God made you a sprinter, don't punish yourself for not keeping up with the person endowed for long-distance running. No matter how hard you work, you won't be a great marathoner. On the other hand, if you are a long, lean marathoner, don't expect to run the world's best 100-meter dash. The ultimate capacity of your heart and lungs, the ability of your blood to carry oxygen, the mix and type of muscle fibers you possess—all these factors and more determine your athletic potential. The good news is this: Whatever your aerobic potential, you can improve it substantially.

Gender and age.

Women athletes have been closing the gap on men for almost three decades now. Among world-class endurance athletes, the difference between the performance of women and men is about 10 percent. In strength events the difference is greater. Women athletes were held back from athletics so long that we probably haven't seen yet what they can really do. I expect to see the gender gap narrow as more and more women enter sports. Gender is a factor in determining ultimate performance in endurance sports, but it is irrelevant for those on the journey of fitness. Age is more significant than gender. People who are sedentary experience a decline in fitness of about 10 percent every decade while those who are moderately active decline at about 5 percent. Here's the good news: People who are active and engage in ongoing fitness programs decline by only 2.5 percent per decade. If you make a long-term commitment to aerobic fitness, you will cut the effects of aging on physical endurance by 75 percent!

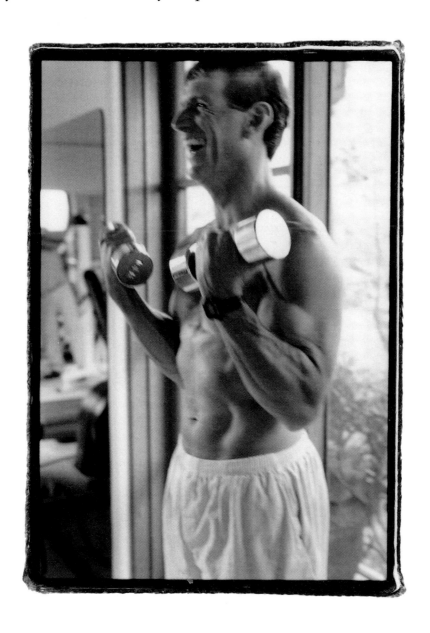

EXERCISE
AND GROW
STRONG

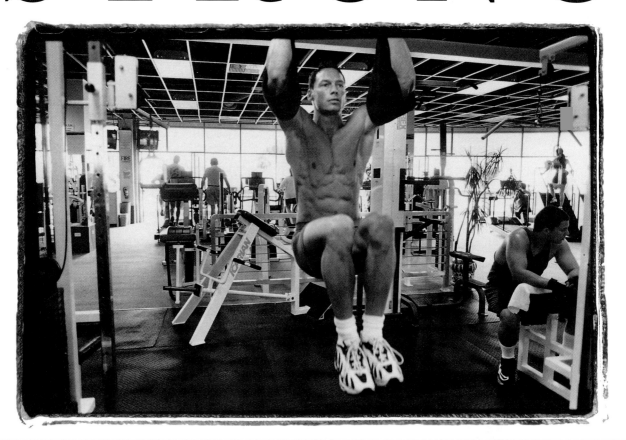

I said earlier that a balanced program achieves both aerobic and muscular fitness. But only a few years ago muscular fitness was not considered important by many experts. Muscular fitness had a bad name for a long time. People associated it with extreme body building, steroids, and a gym culture that valued mass and size over athleticism. Times have changed, and now virtually every fitness expert recognizes the importance of maintaining and building muscle mass. Like aerobic fitness, strength declines with age if we are sedentary. Our bodies grow stronger through our formative years, and our strength peaks when we are about twenty. Unless we exercise, our strength declines slowly and steadily after we pass age twenty; it continues to decline until we reach sixty and then falls off dramatically. However, if we engage in resistance training, our strength does not decline at all. Many competitive weight lifters have achieved their personal best in their mid-forties. In fact, we now know that through resistance training we can achieve significant gains in strength even into our nineties. We are never too old to improve the strength of our muscles.

In chapter six I will give you some specific advice on different types of resistance training routines that have been successful for my clients. But first, there are some basic principles that you should first understand about muscular fitness.

The overload principle.

If you want to improve the strength of any muscle, you must work it hard enough to impose an overload. In technical terms, this means that you have to load a muscle to at least two-thirds of its maximum capacity—if you don't, the muscle won't grow. In the chapter on strength-training workouts I'll give you some tips on how to gauge when you're working

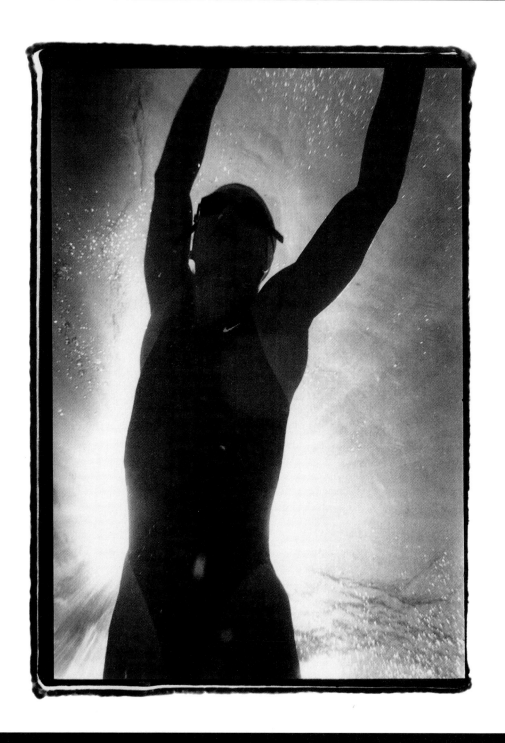

hard enough. As you gain strength, you must continually challenge the muscle, adding more weight or more repetitions to your exercise.

The adaptation principle.

Your body will adapt to the type of resistance training you do. If your resistance program involves heavy weights and few repetitions, you will gain strength but not endurance. If you lift light weights but do many repetitions, you will gain muscular endurance but not strength. If you follow a program somewhere in between these two, you will get mixed results. Some studies indicate that a program that combines high resistance/low repetitions and low resistance/high repetitions is better than taking the middle road.

The variability principle.

The human body will quickly adjust itself to any repetitious exercise routine. If you do the same workout all the time you will make progress at first, then plateau. I change my clients' routines constantly, never doing the same thing twice in a week. The goal is to constantly surprise the body with new and unexpected demands. When you adhere to the variability principle, the result is constant growth and progress.

The balance principle.

Most every muscle in your body works in opposition to another. A good resistance program recognizes that the body is held in dynamic tension by these opposing muscle groups. Exercises for the chest need to be offset by exercises for the upper back, the biceps with the triceps, and so forth. Groups of muscles should also be balanced. The upper body shouldn't be neglected in favor of the lower and vice versa. Bodybuilders sometimes have massive upper bodies but skinny legs, and runners often have beautifully developed legs but poor upper body strength. Always seek balance in your resistance-training program.

Strength training will improve your athletic performance and build muscle that cannot be gained through aerobic exercise. It is quite possible to be in superb aerobic condition while losing important muscle mass. You should always combine aerobic training with strength work—you will be more active and vigorous if you do. If done properly, resistance training will improve your posture and help prevent back injuries. It will strengthen and stabilize the joints in your arms, legs, and shoulders, and it will decrease the chance of injury during aerobic exercise. Resistance training can resculpt your body, adding or maintaining muscle tissue while firming your hips and abdominals.

I began this chapter by saying that exercise enhances both body and soul. People on the journey of fitness often consider aerobic exercise—a long run, for instance—to be a form of meditation, a contemplative act. Resistance training, on the other hand, gives many people a sense of empowerment and vitality. Done together, these two forms of exercise can revitalize you in surprising and powerful ways.

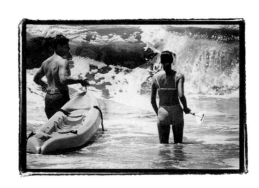

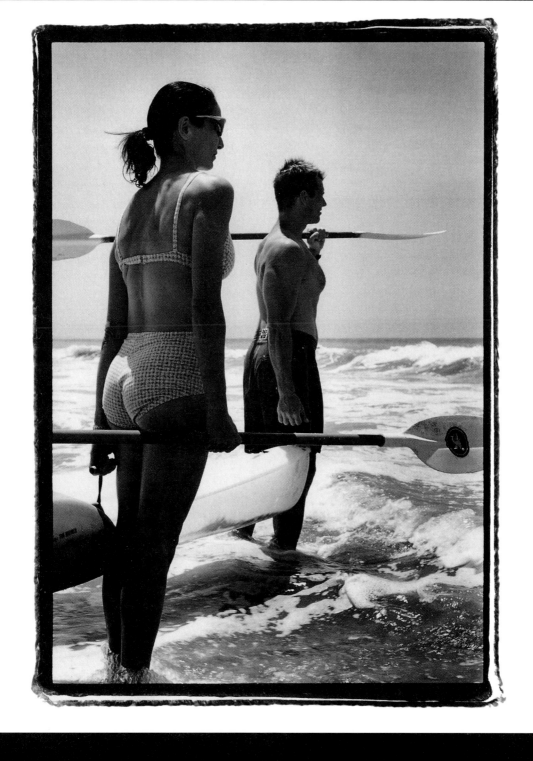

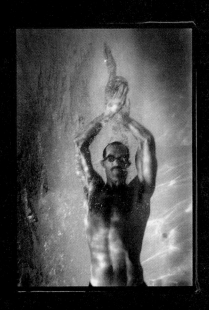

STRENGTH FOR THE JOURNEY

One day a lawyer who represented Sean Penn told me that Sean needed to gain thirty pounds of muscle for his role in a new film, At Close Range. *"Could you help him with that?" he said. "Yes," I replied. A few days later I was training Sean in Los Angeles. The movie was to be filmed on location in Tennessee, and after a few weeks of working out in L. A., Sean asked me if I would go with him. I said, "I'll need more money to do something like that." Sean gave a look that said, "So this is a problem?" The producer called me the next day and asked how much I needed. I took a deep breath and said, "Fifteen hundred a week." Without hesitation he said, "Done!" I quickly added, "Plus expenses." "Done." "And a car?" "Done." I was beginning to like Hollywood.*

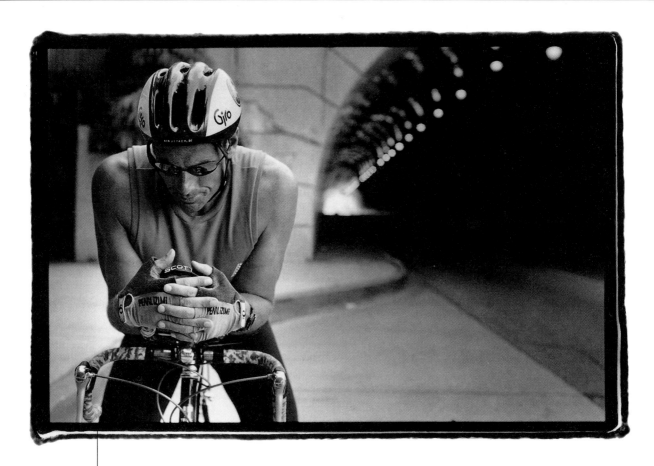

the body adapts

Your body is highly adaptable, and if you
only cycle, for example, you will not achieve
optimum all-around fitness. Unless you are a
competitive athlete it's best to balance your
favorite sport with other activities.

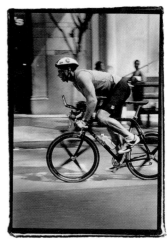

EMPOWER YOURSELF

FOR THE LONG RUN

In this chapter we will look at some specific aerobic-training programs. When it comes to aerobic training, there are an infinite number of possibilities, and I encourage you to use your imagination and growing experience to constantly modify whatever program you decide to pursue. In the last chapter, I talked about the importance of variety in any fitness program but I want to emphasize it again, because it is at the heart of my exercise philosophy. Always keep in mind that whatever program you perform on a given day, that program will only work a certain set of muscles in a very specific way. Unless you are a competitive athlete training for an individual sport, I recommend you constantly change your regimen. If you cycle, for example, your muscles, tendons, ligaments, nerves, and cardiovascular system will adapt in a very specialized manner to that particular exercise. However, if you constantly vary your workouts, you will not only avoid boredom, you will achieve a higher level of overall fitness. Your body is marvelously adaptable, and you can train it to become a specialist or a generalist. If you are a competitive athlete, you will want to be a specialist.

But if you seek fitness, the advantages of being a generalist are many. A generalist practices several aerobic sports. Generalists are more versatile, less prone to repetitive-use injuries, and more apt to stick with a long-term program.

How much improvement can you expect from aerobic exercise? The results will vary depending on your base level of fitness. The more out of shape you are, the more dramatic your improvement will be. People who are sedentary can improve their fitness level by 30 percent while seasoned athletes may improve by only 5 percent. But these figures are deceptive. The subjective improvements are much greater. Scientific studies on aerobic fitness usually focus on the body's ability to utilize and transport oxygen, a measurement referred to as VO_2 max. While this is a useful measurement, it doesn't say much about real-life fitness. A gain in VO_2 max of 30 percent is certainly significant, but in the end it is only a measure of genetic potential and your progress toward it. A more meaningful measure for most people is called "submaximal capacity." This refers to a person's ability to continue for indefinite periods activities that were once fatiguing or even impossible. Expect dramatic improvements in your submaximal capacity.

So how do you get on the road to aerobic fitness? Here are a few suggestions that might help you get started.

Make a commitment.

This is the first step. There is no use talking about it—or just reading this book—unless you decide to take action. I train some of the busiest and most successful people in the world, and they manage to find time for health. You can, too.

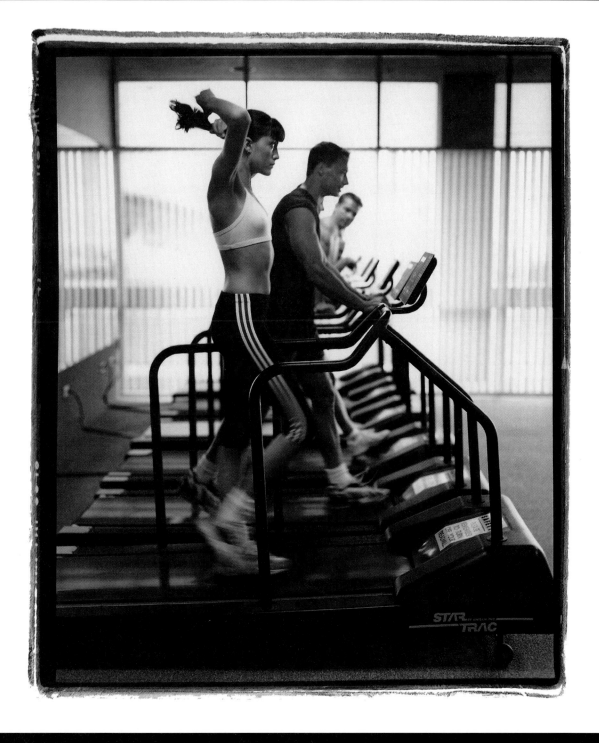

149

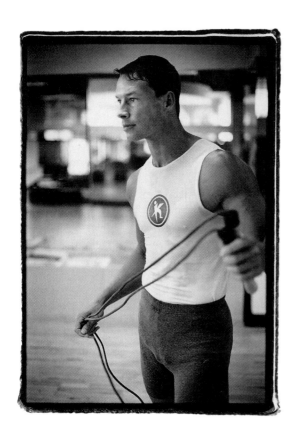

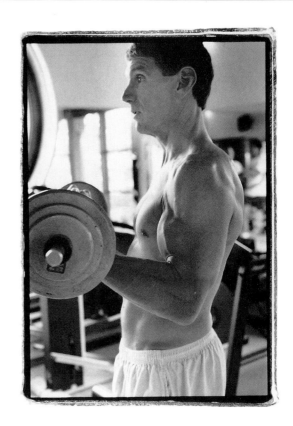

Get a physical.

This is particularly important if you haven't exercised in a while, or if your are over age thirty-five. Exercise is not hazardous, but it's a good idea to establish a health baseline. Items you may want to have checked are your cardiovascular function, body fat, blood cholesterol, and triglycerides. If you can see a physician who specializes in sports medicine, all the better. Many physicians are themselves unfit and not good sources of advice on the benefits of physical activity. Use your judgment.

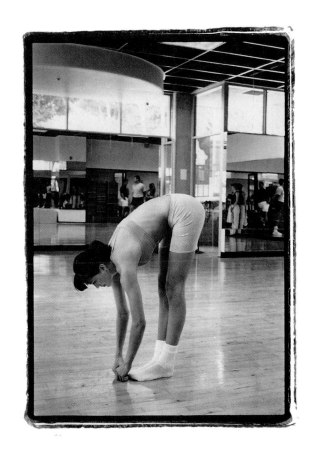

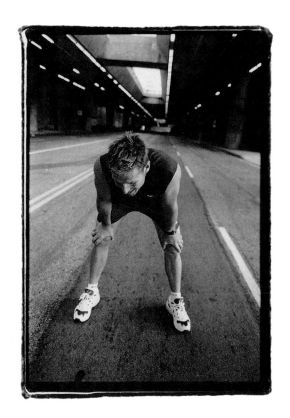

Pay attention to injuries.

If you have an old injury, or any physical problem that causes pain, choose an aerobic program that will avoid making that injury worse. Don't take the macho approach and try to work through the pain.

Pick a specific time and place.

If you live a regimented life, a nine-to-five job, for example, decide what time is best for you (before or after work, at lunch) and stick with it.

Change your priorities.

Make aerobic fitness a top priority in your life. What is more important than living long and living well? What good is success without health?

Start slowly.

Don't be concerned about what others are doing and don't be competitive. It takes time to achieve aerobic fitness—in fact, it is a lifelong process! Give yourself a break and ease into your program.

Be consistent.

No aerobic program will work if you don't stick with it. Exercise should become a regular part of your life, like eating and sleeping. If you are inconsistent, the results you achieve will be minimal. Fitness is gained slowly but lost quickly.

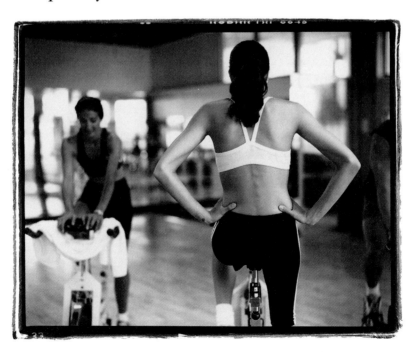

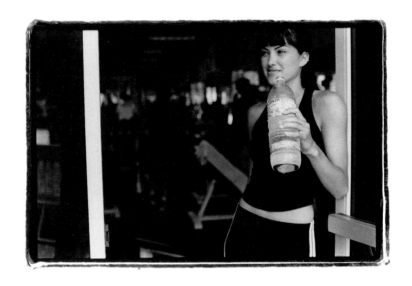

Set realistic goals.

Seek balance in your aerobic work. If you set your goals too high, you will be disappointed and vulnerable to injury. If you set your goals too low, you won't make good progress.

Find a workout partner.

A workout partner has been called the poor man's personal trainer. A good partner will call you if you don't show up to run, encourage you when you're out of energy, and give you a hard time when you slack off! Aerobic workouts are always more fun if they are social occasions.

Dress appropriately.

You don't need anything fancy for aerobic work, but you do need good shoes, especially if you plan to run. I recommend that you buy your shoes at a store that has trained, knowledgeable salespeople. You can work out in whatever is comfortable for you, but avoid clothing that doesn't breath. There are all kinds of sport-specific, high-tech apparel on the market, but some people still prefer old-fashioned cotton (at least for warm weather workouts). The choice is yours.

Reward yourself.

When you reach milestones, celebrate. Shop for a new suit or dress and show off those lost inches. Buy yourself a small gift or do something special.

Every aerobic exercise session—no matter what activity you choose—should start with a period of warming up and stretching. A brief warm-up will increase your body temperature, respiration, and heart rate, and will help to prevent injuries. I usually begin with a few minutes of easy stretching. I reserve any intense stretching for later in the workout, when the muscles, tendons, and ligaments are thoroughly warm. When your body is cold, it's particularly important not to do any ballistic stretching. Ballistic stretching is the kind that involves bouncing or jerking of the muscle. This kind of stretching can result in injury. Start off with some nice, slow dynamic stretches. Think of a cat, when it slowly arches its back and stretches its legs, or a T'ai Chi master, leading a group of students in long, slow, graceful movements. After a few minutes of loosening up your muscles and joints, gradually begin your workout, building up intensity as your temperature rises. After your workout, be sure to cool down slowly. A cooldown is just as important as a warm-up. Some studies suggest that a good cooldown will help prevent cramping, soreness, and other problems. It will also help your body to move waste products (like lactic acid and carbon dioxide) out of your muscles and bloodstream.

Feel free to choose any form of aerobic exercise you like. No one mode of exercise is best, except the one *you* want to do. The same benefits accrue no matter what you choose. When I train Madonna, I rotate the aerobic exercises we do through a cycle that includes running, cycling, in-line skating, aerobic circuit training, treadmill, VersaClimber, and Lifecycle. But what if you're not in the same condition as Madonna? You might want to start by simply walking.

Walking

Walking is an excellent aerobic exercise. You don't have to learn any new skills, own any exotic equipment, or drive to a specialized facility. Many sports physicians and fitness researchers think walking is the best way to start building aerobic fitness, and several of them have suggested similar programs. The following is a six-month program for people who are out of shape. At the end of the six months, you can elect to continue walking as your main aerobic exercise, or you can move on to more strenuous activities. Walking is something you can do for a lifetime.

If you plan to walk, invest in a pair of walking shoes. A good walking shoe is different from a running shoe. The proper shoe will help prevent foot and ankle problems and help cushion your stride so that your lower back doesn't take a beating. A walking shoe is more flexible than a running shoe and has a reinforced heel counter, which helps to locate your ankle firmly. When you walk, your heel takes more of a beating than when you run, so you will need more cushioning in this area. Don't let an inexperienced sales clerk sell you a running shoe. The biomechanics of walking are much different from those of running.

WALKING PROGRAM FOR BEGINNERS

(Start with this program if you have been completely sedentary.)

WEEK	1	2	3	4	5	6	7	8
Warm-up Time (min)	5-7	5-7	5-7	5-7	5-7	5-7	5-7	5-7
Miles to Walk	0.5	0.6	0.75	0.75	0.8	0.9	1.0	1.0
Pace in Miles per Hour	2.0	2.0	2.5	2.5	2.5	3.0	3.0	3.0
Heart Rate (% of max)	50-60	50-60	60	60	60-70	60-70	60-70	60-70
Duration of Walk (min)	15	18	18	18	19.5	22	20	20
Cooldown Time (min)	5-7	5-7	5-7	5-7	5-7	5-7	5-7	5-7
Walks per Week	5	5	5	5	5	5	5	5

WEEK	9	10	11	12	13	14	15	16
Warm-up Time (min)	5-7	5-7	5-7	5-7	5-7	5-7	5-7	5-7
Miles to Walk	1.0	1.1	1.25	1.5	1.5	1.75	1.75	1.75
Pace in Miles per Hour	2.5	2.5	2.5	2.5	3.0	3.0	3.0	3.5
Heart Rate (% of max)	60-70	60-70	60-70	60-70	60-70	60-70	70	70
Duration of Walk (min)	24	27	30	36	30	30	26	26
Cooldown Time (min)	5-7	5-7	5-7	5-7	5-7	5-7	5-7	5-7
Walks per Week	5	5	5	5	5	5	5	5

WEEK	17	18	19	20	21	22	23	24
Warm-up Time (min)	5-7	5-7	5-7	5-7	5-7	5-7	5-7	5-7
Miles to Walk	1.75	1.8	1.8	2.0	2.0	2.0	2.25	2.25
Pace in Miles per Hour	3.5	4.0	4.0	3.5	4.0	4.5	4.5	4.5
Heart Rate (% of max)	70	70	70	70	70	70	70-80	70-80
Duration of Walk (min)	26	27	27	34	30	27	30	30
Cooldown Time (min)	5-7	5-7	5-7	5-7	5-7	5-7	5-7	5-7
Walks per Week	5	5	5	5	5	5	5	5

Calories Expended for a Brisk 30-Minute Walk/3.5 miles per hour

BODY WEIGHT	95 lb	125 lb	155 lb	185 lb	215 lb	245 lb
CALORIES BURNED	85	114	140	158	195	222

4 miles per hour

BODY WEIGHT	95 lb	125 lb	155 lb	185 lb	215 lb	245 lb
CALORIES BURNED	97	130	140	168	220	250

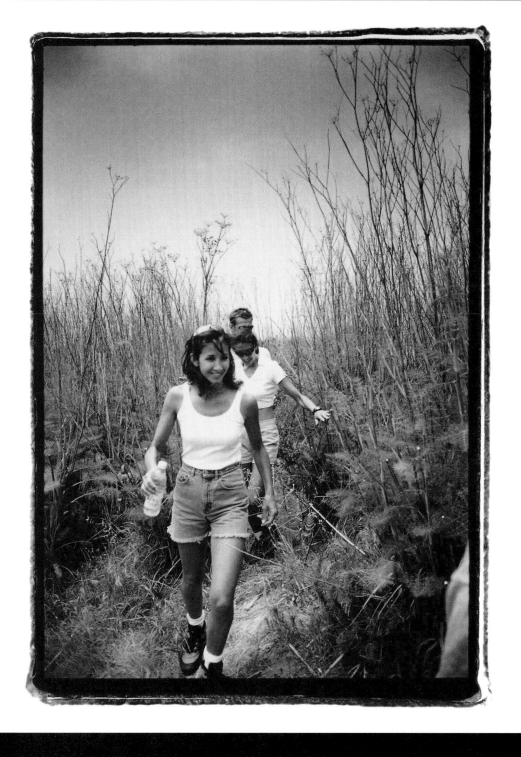

Running

Running, like walking, has the advantage of not needing much equipment and is something you can do almost anywhere and anytime. You do, however, need a good pair of running shoes. Running shoes should be well padded, flexible around the ball of the foot, and carefully fitted. There are many excellent shoes on the market. Find one that is well suited to the idiosyncrasies of your feet and your style of running. A good sports store and salesperson will help you pick a model that is appropriate to your running style and the unique way your foot hits the ground (i.e., your footstrike). Again, you can wear whatever clothing is most comfortable for you, but I recommend apparel that is loose fitting, breathes well, and does not bind. Women will want to wear a supportive jogging bra.

If you started with the walking program above, you may want to begin by alternating your run with periods of walking. The rule of thumb for beginners is to walk two minutes and run two minutes, gradually increasing the amount of time you spend running. Many people get discouraged when they start running because they start out too aggressively. You shouldn't be running so fast that you can't carry on a conversation with your workout partner. Go easy on yourself. Running should be a joy. In my opinion, running provides psychological and spiritual benefits that walking does not. I'm not dogmatic about that, but in general I think it's true. "Runner's high" is a real phenomenon. The euphoria that runners feel keeps them coming back time and again, seeking that "zone" where the world's cares melt away in the rhythm of their measured breaths and regular strides. Work your way gradually to the point where you reach a kind of homeostasis, a point at which it seems you could go on forever. It will take some time to get there, but look forward to it and be patient. Slowly work your way up to where you can run continuously for half an hour. It may take you several weeks or months to accomplish this. If you feel strong and want to achieve higher levels of fitness, work your way up to an hour. To avoid injuries and burnout, never increase your mileage by more than 10 percent per week. Set aside at least one day a week to rest. If you are a new runner, rest two days a week. Your body needs time to recover from the stresses of running.

As with the walking program I have outlined above, keep your heart rate in the 60 to 70 percent of maximum range. Warm up slowly. Vary the intensity of your run by varying your pace. If you are wearing a heart-rate monitor, it will be easy to keep yourself in the aerobic zone. One way to assure an adequate warm-up is to start off walking, then jogging, then running (and then reverse the process for your cooldown). When you run, keep your upper body relaxed and your abdominal muscles pulled in slightly. Pay attention to your posture. If you have a workout partner, have him or her watch you run and point out any gross problems. If your back is arched, for example, you may experience back or hip problems.

CALORIES CONSUMED AT JOGGING PACE
(Per 1/2 hour @ 10 min/mile pace)

Body Weight	95 lb	125 lb	155 lb	185 lb	215 lb	245 lb
Calories Consumed	215	285	350	420	490	555

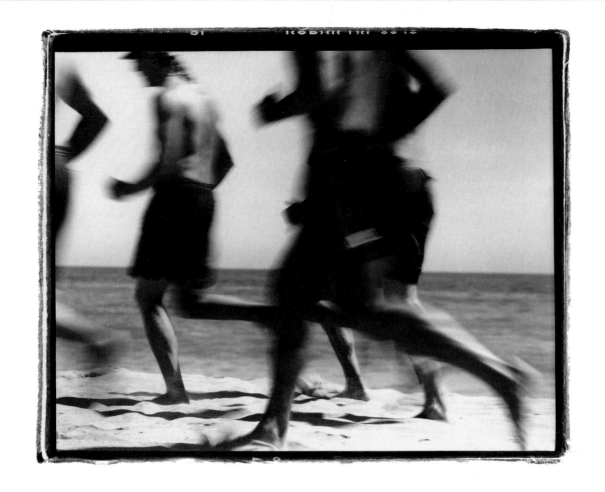

SPEED AND DISTANCE AT DIFFERENT PACES

PACE	1/4 Mile	1/2 Mile	1 Mile
Slow Jog	3 minutes	6 minutes	12 minutes
Jog	1.25 minutes	2.5 minutes	10 minutes
Run	2 minutes	4 minutes	8 minutes
Fast Run	1.5 minutes	3 minutes	6 minutes

BASIC PROGRAM

FOR BEGINNING RUNNERS - JOG/WALK CYCLE

WEEK							
1	2	3	4	5	6	7	8
Jog 40 seconds	Jog 1 minute	Jog 2 minutes	Jog 4 minutes	Jog 6 minutes	Jog 8 minutes	Jog 10 minutes	Jog 12 minutes
Walk 1 minute	Walk 1 minute	Walk 1 minute	Walk 1 minute	Walk 1 minute	Walk 2 minutes	Walk 2 minutes	Walk 2 minutes
CYCLES PER WORKOUT							
9	8	6	4	3	2	2	2
DAYS PER WEEK							
5 days	5 days	5 days	5 days	5 days	5 days	5 days	5 days

BASIC PROGRAM
FOR INTERMEDIATE RUNNERS - JOG/WALK CYCLE

JOG/WALK CYCLE	Run 1 mile	Run 1 mile	Run 1 mile	Run 1 mile	Run 1 mile	Run 1.5 mile	Run 1.5 miles	Run 1 mile
	Walk 5 minutes	Walk 5 minutes	Walk 5 minutes	Walk 5 minutes	Walk 5 minutes	Walk 7 minutes	Walk 7 minutes	Walk 7 minutes
PACE IN MINUTES	12 minutes	11 minutes	10.5 minutes	10 minutes	9.5 minutes	13.5 minutes	13 minutes	8 & 8.5 minutes
	-	-	-	-	2	2	2	2
DAYS PER WEEK	5 days	5 days	5 days	5 days	5 days	5 days	5 days	5 days

BASIC PROGRAM
FOR ADVANCED RUNNERS

MONTH 1	20 miles per week
MONTH 2	25 miles per week
MONTH 3	30 miles per week
MONTH 4	35 miles per week
MONTH 5	40 miles per week
MONTH 6	45 miles per week

- Use a 4 or 5 days-per-week schedule
- Vary mileage and terrain
- Do one long run per week, but not more than 1/3 of total weekly mileage
- Last 20% should be intervals or run at a faster pace

Cycling

Cycling is an excellent aerobic exercise for people of all fitness levels. One of its chief advantages is that it is low impact—unlike running—while still offering a high level of intensity. If you have an injury that might make running uncomfortable, cycling may be a good choice for you. Cycling is also a good complement to walking, because it works primarily the front of the thighs (the quadriceps) while walking works mostly the back of the legs (the hamstrings). Unlike walking and running, however, cycling requires some expensive equipment. At minimum you will need a bicycle, helmet, sunglasses, and cycling shorts—you may also want a pair of cycling shoes. Cycling also requires a few skills. You need to know some basic technique (how to shift, brake, corner, and climb) and enough about the mechanics of the bicycle to maintain it properly, and change a flat if necessary. For some people, a bike's mechanical sophistication and maintenance needs are an asset. There is satisfaction in riding and maintaining a fine machine, and many cyclists consider a good bicycle a work of art.

The two basic choices in bicycles are mountain bikes and road bikes. Each has its own advantages. A mountain bike gives you the freedom to ride dirt roads and trails, and the benefits of ultra-low gearing, rugged construction, and an upright comfortable riding position. A road bike offers light weight, fast handling, low rolling resistance, and more speed (on pavement) for your effort. Both types of bikes have their devotees. If you're a novice, you will probably feel more comfortable on a mountain bike. If you buy a mountain bike but ride mostly on the street, have your dealer install a set of street or "combination" tires. There is no sense in pushing around a set of wide

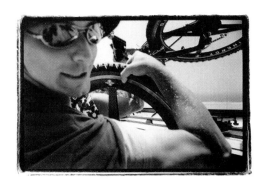

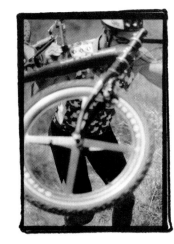

choose your sport

Cycling is just one of many possible
aerobic exercises. It is a low-impact, high-
intensity sport that offers many benefits.

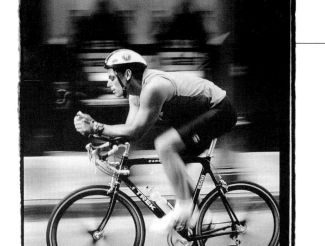

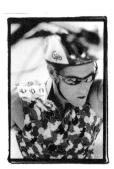

knobby tires on pavement—they handle poorly, and they're noisy and have high rolling resistance. The rule of thumb for buying a bicycle is to get the best one you can afford. Top quality bikes have better components and are generally lighter in weight. Buy a good quality helmet and wear it. Eighty-five percent of fatal head injuries suffered in bicycle accidents could have been prevented by wearing a helmet.

When you go shopping for a bicycle take a knowledgeable friend with you, or go to a shop with a reputation for serving hard-core cyclists. Many people ride bikes that are the wrong size or are poorly set up. It is vital that someone who knows what he is doing helps you choose the proper saddle and sets the height for you, adjusts the rise and reach of the handlebars, and positions the brake levers and shifters to fit your hands and fingers. Experienced cyclists are fanatical about how their bikes are set up because they know a quarter-inch difference in seat height can mean ruin for their knees or a drop in cycling efficiency. Have a fanatic help you adjust your bike—it will pay big dividends!

Vary your cycling on a daily basis. On Mondays, for example, you could begin by taking a thirty-minute ride on flat terrain at an easy to moderate pace. On Tuesdays you could include a little hill climbing on your route; Wednesdays cycle at a fast pace for the second half of your ride; Thursdays do intervals; Friday or Saturday take an extra-long ride. Try to keep your heart rate up in the training zone for most of your ride. Riding downhill for most of your route might be fun, but not much of a workout!

Swimming

If you have easy access to a pool, swimming is an excellent form of aerobic exercise. Swimming works the entire body and is a sustained form of activity that keeps the heart rate up continuously. Water supports your body, making swimming a zero-impact sport. Swimming is probably the best form of exercise for people who have injuries, particularly back problems, arthritis, or joint diseases. The only downside is that it is not as effective as land-based activities in burning fat. Because water is an efficient thermal conductor, it dissipates body heat and doesn't raise your core temperature as much as other activities. You'll burn many calories while you're swimming, but few after you quit. Ocean or lake swimming is great fun. If you swim in a natural setting, away from people, lifeguards, or the security of a readily accessible poolside, use good judgment. A pair of swim fins or a kickboard will provide a margin of safety.

If you swim regularly in a chlorinated pool, you'll want a pair of goggles. In addition, most regular swimmers prefer Speedos, or a similar swimsuit for aerobic work. Baggies, or surfer-style trunks, are not as comfortable because they tend to bunch up in your crotch. If you'd rather die than be seen in a pair of Speedos, buy the trimmest pair of trunks you feel comfortable in. There are a variety of accessories on the market for swimmers, including fins, hand paddles, pull buoys, and kickboards. If any of these devices seem fun or effective, try them out. Hand paddles will increase the intensity of your upper body workout (which is good), but don't use them for every workout—you can strain your shoulders if you do.

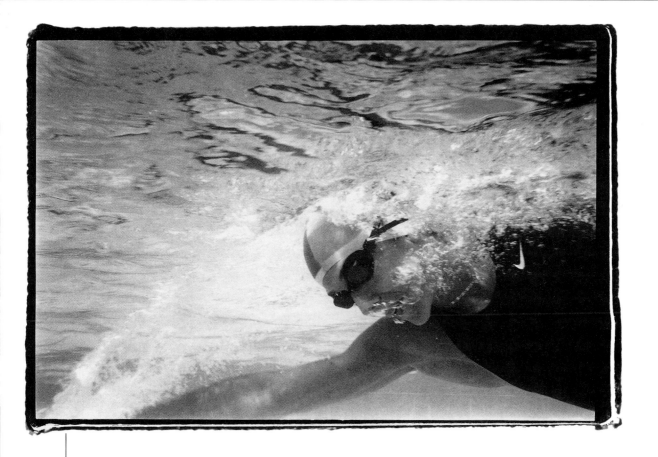

do what you enjoy

Swimming is an excellent form of exercise
that works the entire body, is easy on the
joints, and is particularly good for people
with injuries.

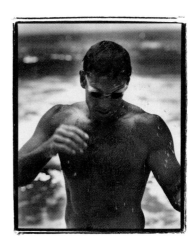

BASIC PROGRAM

FOR BEGINNING SWIMMERS (After 8 weeks design your own program—do what you enjoy!)

WEEK	Mon, Wed Aerobic Work (rest at midpoint if necessary)						
1	2	3	4	5	6	7	8
15 min Easy Pace	15 min Easy Pace	20 min Easy Pace	20 min Moderate Pace	25 min Moderate Pace	30 min Moderate Pace	30 min Moderate Pace	35 min Moderate Pace
Tues, Thurs Intervals							
3 4-min Intervals Moderate Pace	2 5-min Intervals Moderate Pace	3 5-min Intervals Moderate Pace	2 8-min Intervals Hard Pace	3 7-min Intervals Hard Pace	2 12-min Intervals Hard Pace	3 9-min Intervals Hard Pace	2 15-min Intervals Hard Pace
Friday Overdistance							
20 min Easy Pace	20 min Easy Pace	25 min Easy Pace	30 min Moderate Pace	35 min Moderate Pace	40 min Moderate Pace	45 min Moderate Pace	50 min Moderate Pace
Sat-Sun							
Rest or Easy Waterplay	Rest or Easy Waterplay	Rest or Easy Waterplay	Rest or Easy Waterplay	Rest or Easy Waterplay	Rest or Easy Waterplay	Rest or Easy Waterplay	Rest or Easy Waterplay

CALORIES CONSUMED WHILE SWIMMING
(Per 1/2 Hour)

Body Weight	95 lb	125 lb	155 lb	185 lb	215 lb	245 lb
Calories Consumed Easy Pace	130	170	210	250	295	333
Calories Consumed Hard Pace	215	285	350	420	490	555

In-Line Skating

In-line skating is enormously popular in Southern California where I live and is the most rapidly growing aerobic sport in the nation. In-line skating works the legs, hips and hip flexors, and the butt. If you keep up a good pace, it is one of the best cardiovascular exercises you can do. It can also be one of the most fun. You can go forward, backward, freestyle, or speed skate and enjoy a freedom of movement that is unknown in most sports. Hard-core in-line skaters think it is the most exhilarating aerobic exercise on the planet. There is one downside, however: This is one sport that requires skill. Unless you have an experienced friend who can teach you how to skate, you may want to take lessons or attend a workshop. You'll probably pick up the basic motions fairly quickly, but some skills take time to master—not the least of which is stopping! In-line skates have rudimentary brakes that are counterintuitive to use. Any speed sport that considers stopping to be an advanced skill is one that must be taken seriously!

Like cycling, in-line skating is an equipment-intensive sport. It's not cheap getting started. You will need a good-quality pair of skates; knee, elbow, and wrist guards; and a helmet. Don't take the macho (i.e., dumb) approach and skip the safety equipment. Nearly 200,000 in-line skaters a year make an unplanned trip to the nearest hospital emergency room. It is easy to get going very fast, very quickly, and many novices end up making involuntary use of a curb or a tree to stop. If you are wearing the right equipment, your chances of sustaining a serious injury are greatly diminished. Be prepared to spend serious money. If you buy your equipment one piece at a time, buy the safety paraphernalia first and avoid the temptation to try out those shiny new skates without a

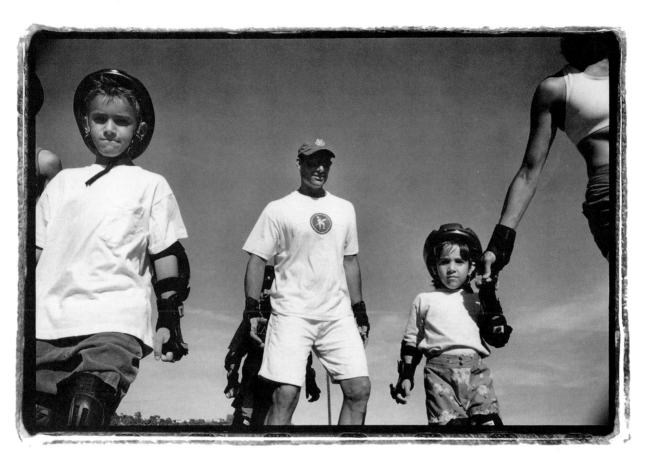

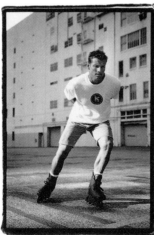

get outdoors

Working out on a treadmill inside a gym is okay, but exercising outdoors is much more exhilarating. In-line skating is great fun and an excellent way to get your aerobic exercise.

helmet or wrist guards. As with a bike, seek out a good retailer, one who knows the equipment thoroughly and will spend the time to fit you correctly. Don't buy equipment from anyone who doesn't skate. It's like getting advice on a tennis racket from someone who doesn't play the game.

OTHER AEROBIC SPORTS

Cross-Country Skiing

Competitive cross-country skiers are generally considered the most aerobically fit endurance athletes in the world. Cross-country skiing is a superb form of cardiovascular exercise that also builds muscular strength. It is a low-impact sport that works mostly the legs, but also involves major muscles in the upper back, shoulders, and arms. That's the good news. The bad news: You need snow! Cross-country skiing is a seasonal sport—except, perhaps, in Minnesota. Cross-country ski machines, like a NordicTrack, can provide most of the benefits of skiing in snow, but without the fresh air and nice view. It takes a while to learn the motions involved in using a stationary machine, so don't get discouraged before you get the hang of it.

Paddleboarding

Paddleboarding is one of my favorite aerobic sports. I live a few hundred yards from the Pacific Ocean, so this form of exercise is a practical one for me. The ocean or any large body of water is suitable for paddleboarding. Typically, I combine this activity with one that works primarily the legs. Paddleboarding is an upper body exercise that works the arms, shoulders, chest, and back. Paddleboards are larger and less expensive than surfboards and require little ancillary equipment except swim trunks, a rash guard for your chest, and sunscreen.

Rowing

Rowing is a high-intensity sport that works your entire body, especially your legs, upper and lower back, shoulders, and arms. Competitive rowers are among the best-conditioned aerobic athletes in the world. If you plan to row on water, however, you will need to live within range of a rowing club or other facility. More likely, you will do your rowing on a machine at a health club or purchase a stationary rowing machine for home use. Form is crucial in rowing, because of the potential for lower-back injuries from poor technique. An instructional video, trainer, or coach can show you how to do it right.

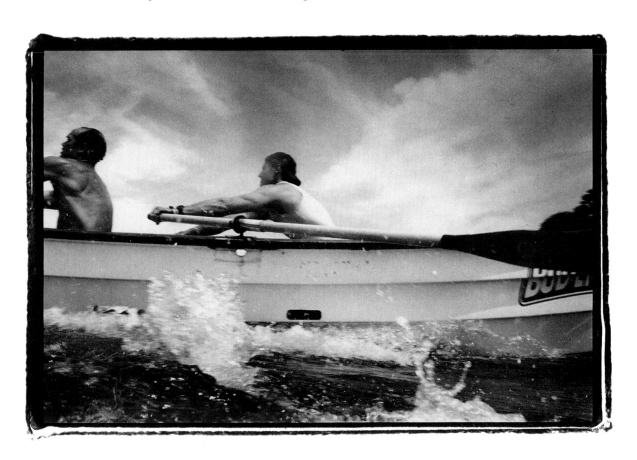

Spinning

Spinning is a high-intensity, high-energy form of aerobic cycling that uses a stationary bicycle. Spinning classes use a special type of stationary bike that is set up to simulate a road bike. Spinning bikes have racing seats, often have clip-in pedals (the kind that require special shoes and cleats), and handlebars that resemble the "aero" bars on racing bikes. An instructor leads the class for fifty minutes of choreographed riding. Spinning works the quads, hamstrings, buttocks, and lower back. Spinning classes can be tremendous fun, and the enthusiastic support of fellow classmates can carry you to new heights of exertion. There are classes for people of all levels, but spinning is particularly popular with the real hammer heads.

Step Aerobics/Aerobic Dance

Aerobics classes at gyms, health clubs, Y's, and community centers are ubiquitous these days. An aerobics class can give you a good cardiovascular workout and help strengthen your lower body muscles. There can be some benefit to your upper body and abdominals, depending on how the class is taught. Step aerobics uses your body weight to increase the cardiovascular load and raise your heart rate. If you're unselfconscious and like to dance, dance aerobics class can be fun and is potentially a great form of exercise. If you choose step or dance aerobics, shop around and see what class suits you best. It's important to find one that matches your level of fitness and coordination. The skill of aerobics teachers varies considerably. Seek an instructor who is certified by an aerobics association.

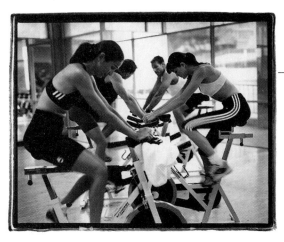

It doesn't matter whether you spin or take an aerobics class, or do both. Enjoy what you do, and if you get tired of one activity, try another.

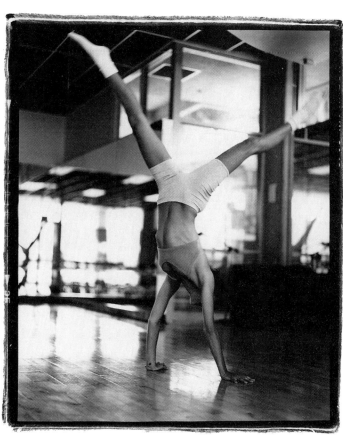

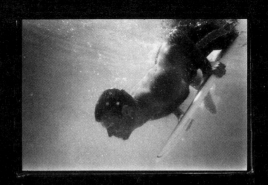

P O W E R   F O R   L I F E

I traveled all over the world with Sean Penn for four years. I built him up or pared him down, depending on the demands of each role he played—big and bulky for At Close Range, *lean and mean for* Dead Man Walking, *and somewhere in between for* Colors. *While I was working with him, I met Madonna. She would join us for workouts, both before and after her marriage to Sean. I helped her find a personal trainer of her own. After Madonna and Sean divorced, she called me one day and asked if I would take her on as a client. She wanted me six days a week, three hours a day. I called Sean. "Is it okay?" He had no objection.*

WORK OUT AND GROW STRONG

Strength training is an essential part of fitness for both men and women. When I first started at Gold's Gym, there were many women bodybuilders who worked out there, but the general public still considered weight training an essentially masculine activity. The persistent myth was that women who lifted weights would become overly muscular and end up looking like men. It *is* possible for women to become overly muscular, but not from lifting weights. Unless women take steroids or human growth hormone, they simply do not develop the heavy musculature of male bodybuilders (and neither will most men!). What women *will* gain from strength training is a toned and beautifully sculpted body. Madonna's physique is testimony to the effectiveness of weight training for women. Unfortunately, the misconception still persists in some circles that strength training is of limited value for women. This is a sexist attitude. Any physical regimen that is healthy for

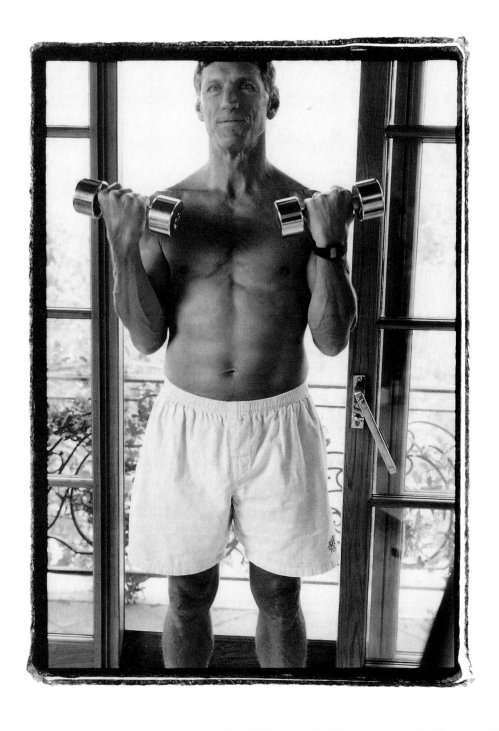

men is also healthy for women. In fact, the benefits of strength training for women are essential to long-term health. An intense program of aerobics without strength training can actually increase the risk of osteoporosis. And for postmenopausal women, weight training is essential to the maintenance of bone density, strength, and balance.

Strength training, like aerobic training, can be done in an infinite variety of ways. There are literally thousands of combinations of exercises you can do. People who have been training for years are still adding new routines, refinements, and variations to their strength-training regimens. I'm learning more all the time and constantly adding to my own repertoire. Consequently, there is no reason to become bored or stale in your workouts. It's a good thing that fitness is a lifelong process, because it takes a lifetime to explore all the possibilities! I encourage you to read about strength training while you are on the road to fitness, so you can add knowledge and new information to your workouts on a continuing basis. There is a large body of literature on the subject written by scientists, bodybuilders, Olympic coaches, and others. A good addition to your fitness library would be a reference book (there are several) that illustrates the hundreds of strength-training exercises traditionally used by athletes, and the correct form for each. This chapter will introduce you to the basics.

Strength training requires the use of various kinds of equipment. There are strength-training exercises that use only body weight for resistance, such as push-ups and pull-ups, but the most effective regimens always use some sort of apparatus. In general, there are two major categories of strength-training equipment: machines and free weights. Machines come in an astonishing variety and are made by a wide range of manufacturers including Nautilus, Cybex, Universal, Paramount, Hammer Strength, Lifecircuit, and others. Most machines involve pushing or pulling a bar or handles with your feet, legs, or hands. Many machines are designed to be used while seated on an adjustable cushion or backrest while moving, via cables or cams, a variable weight stack or hydraulic piston.

"Machines are easier to use for beginners than free weights, because they require less technique."

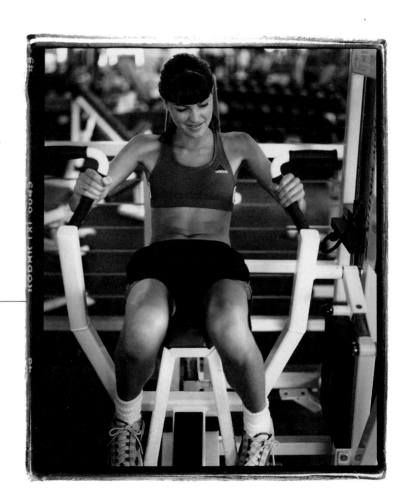

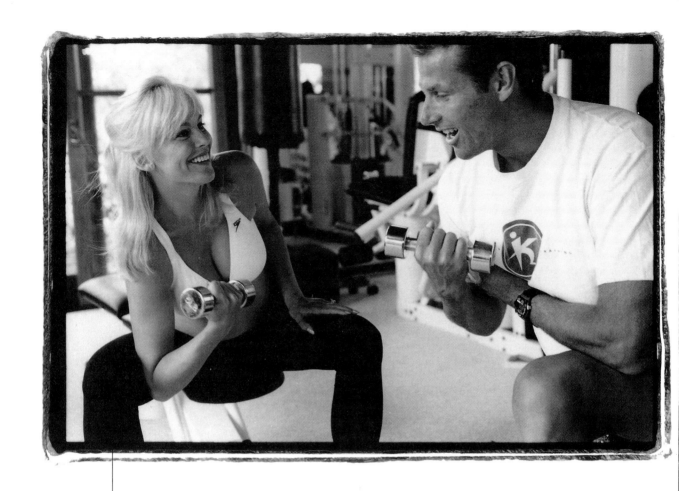

maternity workout

Maintaining fitness while you're pregnant is healthy for you
and your baby, too. Eloise DeJoria worked out until a few
days before she gave birth. A healthy baby is only one benefit
of a healthy lifestyle.

Some strength-training machines provide what is called an *isokinetic* workout. Opinions vary, but some trainers believe that an isokinetic workout is superior to other forms. The Nautilus machine was the first of the isokinetic devices to come on the market. This kind of machine puts the muscle under a different type of load than free weights do. Because your arms and legs act like levers when you lift a free weight, you have the least leverage at the beginning of the movement, and the most at the end. This means that your muscle works the hardest at the beginning of the movement, and less as the motion progresses. An isokinetic machine compensates for changes in leverage by increasing the resistance through the full range of motion and maintaining the same intensity for the entire contraction. Theoretically, at least, this leads to strengthening the muscle through its complete range of motion.

Machines are easier to use for beginners than free weights, because they require less technique. Your range of motion and posture is limited by the geometry and mechanics of the machine (so you don't have to worry too much about form), and if you lose your grip, the weight stack won't fall on your toe (i.e., they're safer). It's also easier to change resistance levels with a machine than with free weights. Machines allow you to get a workout done more quickly if you're in a hurry. A line of machines at a gym provides a ready-made series of quick-and-easy exercises. Machines are also good for solo workouts (many free-weight exercises require someone to spot for you). But if you are a beginner and have never used a particular machine (or any machine!), have someone who is experienced help you get started. Don't assume that strength-training machines require no knowledge at all. Sometimes their operation is less than obvious. Many machines have operating instructions and/or graphics attached to them. It's always a good idea to read

"Free-weight exercises more closely resemble every-day, real-life movements."

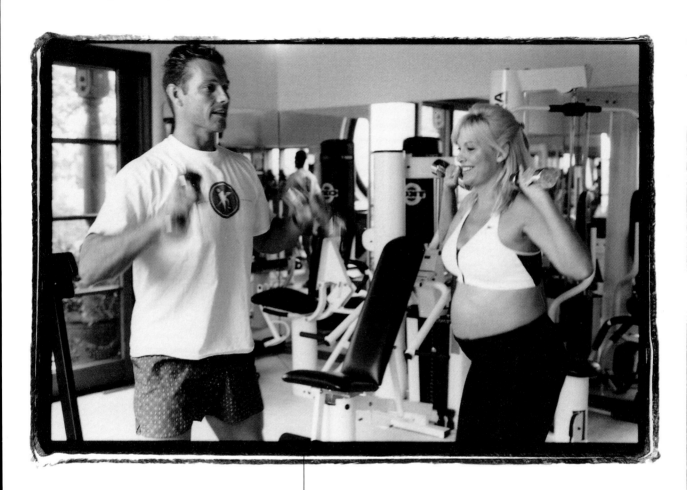

be sensible

Pregnant women should avoid heavy weights and high-impact exercises, but otherwise only a few restrictions apply. Light weights and moderate to high-repetition routines are the sensible approach for pregnant women.

them. Make sure the seat/pad height is correct for you, and any other adjustments (for reach or range of motion, for example) are "dialed in" for your particular body dimensions.

"Free weights" is the generic term for barbells and dumbbells. (If you're a real novice and don't know the difference, barbells are the larger of the two and designed to be gripped with both hands; dumbbells are smaller and gripped with one hand.) A typical gym will have barbells (and weight plates of various sizes to put on them) and dumbbells of different fixed weights. Larger gyms will also have a variety of fixed-weight barbells, as well as other exotic sizes and shapes of bare bars (curved, short, and specialty types). A standard Olympic barbell weighs forty-five pounds bare (without any plates on it). For this reason alone, if your gym doesn't have fixed-weight barbells of lesser weight, you may not want to use them until you've built up some strength. Dumbbells, on the other hand, come in weights as small as two pounds and as heavy (at some gyms) as 200. If you join a gym, have someone show you the types of barbells they have, and their uses. Also, be sure to familiarize yourself with the clamps or locking collars that are used to keep the weight plates from sliding off the bar.

"A good resistance program combines the use of machines and free weights."

Free weights are a form of *isotonic* exercise. In spite of the theoretical advantages of isokinetic work, isotonic exercise remains the overwhelming favorite of serious athletes and bodybuilders. Most gym rats believe that free weights are the best way to produce strength and muscle mass.

Free weights lend themselves to a wider variety of exercises, demand a higher degree of coordination and balance, and can result in greater muscle growth. Free-weight exercises more closely resemble every-day, real-life movements. But there are two main disadvantages to free weights: They require more attention to technique than machines do, and the risk of injury is higher. And it's tough, if not impossible, to learn good free-weight technique without expert instruction. You don't have to be an advanced bodybuilder to use free weights, but I strongly advise beginners to start cautiously, seek advice, and don't use heavy weights at first. In my opinion, a good resistance program combines the use of machines and free weights.

The goal of resistance training, whether with machines or free weights, is to overload the muscle you are working for a sufficient period of time to stimulate growth or improve endurance. In practice this means you need to stress a muscle to at least two-thirds of its maximum strength. There are three basic approaches to weight training, and each has its particular benefit. If you work out with high weights and do only a few repetitions ("reps") of each exercise, you will develop increased strength. If, on the other hand, you work out with low weights but perform many repetitions, you will improve your muscular endurance. A third approach takes the middle road, building both strength and endurance, but without optimizing either.

"Different types of workouts create different chemical reactions in the body."

Lifting high weights recruits the maximum number of muscle fibers at one time and results in the highest possible neurological stimulation of the muscle. Lifting lower weights, but doing more repetitions, utilizes fewer muscle fibers but allows them to cycle on and off, alternating their contractions with brief periods of rest. This stimulates physiological changes that enhance endurance. High-weight/low-repetition workouts strengthen connective tissues (tendons and ligaments) and increase a muscle's ability to generate tension by stimulating the production of *contractile proteins*. Low-weight/high-repetition workouts increase the body's supply of *aerobic enzymes* (another form of protein), and thereby enhance endurance. In other words, different types of workouts create different chemical reactions in the body. If you do only high-weight/low-repetition workouts, your aerobic enzymes will actually decrease, and vice versa. Most people take the middle road, neither lifting high weights nor doing many repetitions. I believe that combining strength and endurance training on alternating days can achieve better results (higher levels of strength and endurance), for those at an intermediate or advanced level of fitness, than trying to combine both goals in a single workout.

"The idea is to constantly 'surprise' the body, forcing it to adapt to new stimuli."

I advise my more experienced clients to vary the number of repetitions they do with every single workout—a high-weight/low-repetition routine on one day, followed by a low-weight/high-repetition one the next. The idea is to constantly "surprise" the body, forcing it to adapt to new stimuli.

The kind of workout you do will depend somewhat on your goals. You can bias your workout in favor of the particular objective you want to accomplish. If your desire is to build maximum strength (if you are a football lineman, for instance) you might want to do more strength work and limit your repetitions to four or six on most days, making sure that the last rep always stresses your muscle to the point of failure. On the other hand, if you are a swimmer or cyclist, you may want to emphasize endurance and do twenty-five repetitions, with the last few reps taking the muscle (or muscle group) close to the point of failure. But since most of us are not professional or competitive athletes, the best workout is a balanced one, incorporating both strength and endurance routines equally. I'm often asked the question, Which is better for building muscular definition? High reps or low? The answer is neither. Low body fat is what gives you definition.

Strength-Endurance Continuum

	Maximum Strength	Strength & Endurance	Maximum Endurance
Sets of each exercise	4 to 6	3 to 4	2 to 3
Repetitions per set	2 to 6	8 to 12	15 to 40
Weight	Heavy	Medium to Heavy	Low to Medium

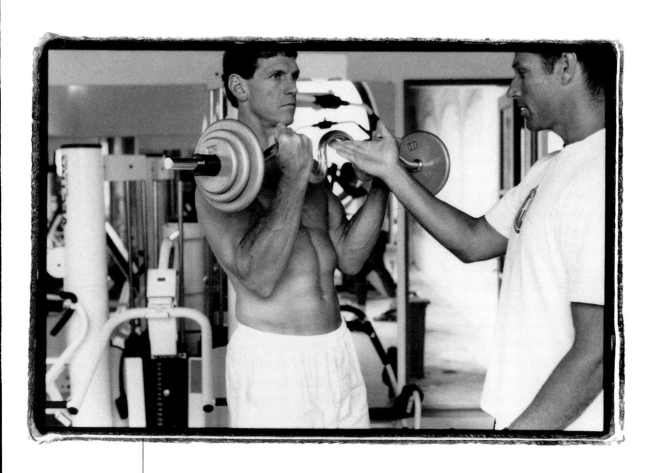

"Your muscles need time to adapt to the new stimulus that weight training provides."

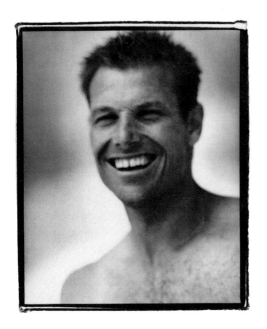

If you work too hard, you'll burn out. Have fun, and you'll stick to your program. Be good to yourself. Give yourself time to adapt and grow.

For beginners I usually recommend starting with ten repetitions of each exercise. This is a good compromise between strength building and endurance. Don't worry about alternating strength and endurance training until you build a base level of fitness. Also, beginners should not work a muscle to the point of failure, but the tenth repetition of an exercise should be strenuous. If you can easily do ten repetitions with a given weight, you should increase the weight. Beginners should always take a few sessions to experiment with each exercise. Give each muscle a gradual wake-up call, rather than jolting it into consciousness by using too much weight or doing too many repetitions. Start with a program of two sessions per week, and do two sets of ten repetitions for each exercise. After two or three weeks, increase your workouts to three sessions per week and three sets of each exercise. As your fitness improves, and your muscles become accustomed to working, your program can be expanded to incorporate more variety and intensity. But remember, when you are starting out, it takes at least forty-eight hours to recover from each weight-training session. Aerobic training is less demanding on the muscles and generally requires less recovery time. Your muscles need time to adapt to the new stimulus that weight training provides. Give them the time they need, and you will get the results you want. If you work too hard, too fast, you will only experience chronic soreness, set yourself up for injury, and get discouraged.

RAY'S RULES
FOR WEIGHT
TRAINING

Warm Up.

As Dr. Brian Sharkey has said, "A warm up is as important for you as it is for your car. During winter months you can't just jump into the old pickup and expect instant performance; you start slowly and avoid overloading the engine until it heats up." A five-to-ten-minute warm-up will increase blood flow to your muscles and reduce the chance of injury.

Stretch.

After you've warmed up, stretch your muscles. Stretching will prepare your joints for work, help maintain (or extend) your muscle's range of motion, and further reduce your chances of injury. Stretch *after* each exercise, too. Stretching the muscle after you work it will elongate the fibers, relieve the stress of the contraction, and reduce soreness.

Use good form.

Good form is essential with free weights. Don't lift weights that are too heavy and try to compensate by using poor form. Keep your body balanced and your back straight. When you are standing upright, keep your feet slightly wider than your shoulders. If you're not sure what good form is for a particular exercise, seek advice.

Use a full range of motion.

You don't want to hyperextend your joints when you work out, but if you use less than a full range of motion, your flexibility will be compromised. A long, lean muscle is the result of good flexibility and working a joint through a *complete* range of motion.

Breathe properly.

Don't hold your breath, except momentarily during the heaviest of lifts. Holding your breath will raise your blood pressure and put your heart under an unnecessary and potentially dangerous load. Breathe out as you push or pull a weight, and breath in as you lower or return it. Blowing air out of your lungs forcefully as you lift will contract your abdomen and stabilize your body. Breathing in while you release the contraction will replenish your lungs with oxygen and release tension. You can inhale through your nose or mouth, but exhale through your mouth.

Be focused.

Isolating the muscle you want to work is essential for good progress. Learn to listen to your body. Focus on your contractions. Where do you feel the strain? If the strain is on an adjacent muscle and not the one you want to work, you're probably using bad form. Pay attention and you will gradually acquire a knowledge of your muscles, their strengths, and weaknesses.

Increase resistance slowly.

Remember that fitness is a lifelong process. You have plenty of time to achieve your goals.

Work with a partner.

If you don't have a trainer, find a workout buddy. Your partner can spot for you, watch your form, encourage you, and give you a hard time when you need it. Having someone spot for you is essential for many free-weight exercises. You can lift more weight safely when someone is standing by to bail you out when you get stuck or tired.

Avoid pain.

Muscle soreness is normal, but pain during a workout is not. If an exercise hurts, stop, evaluate, and try something different.

Rest.

Don't be overzealous. Your body needs rest to recover and adapt to exercise. Insufficient rest will limit your gains.

"Working minor muscle groups is like icing on the cake. But first you have to bake the cake."

There are about 650 muscles in your body, but don't let this fact discourage you—you only need to worry about (approximately) twenty of them! These twenty muscles are organized into six groups. The focus of any good strength-training program is on these major muscle groups. Your own fitness program should include exercises for each. Always resist the temptation to work one group and neglect another. Also, remember to focus on the major muscle groups as the *main emphasis of your routine.* I frequently see people at the gym working minor muscles at the expense of major groups. For example, many gyms have machines that work the leg adductors (inner thighs). This is a perfectly legitimate muscle to work, but it should be considered of secondary importance when compared to working the major functional muscles of the legs—the quadriceps and hamstrings (the seven muscles that cover the front and back of the thighs). Likewise, working the external obliques (the diagonal muscles that run down the sides of your waist) is less important than working the rectus abdominis (the main abdominal muscle that covers the whole front of your lower abdomen). Working minor muscle groups is like icing on the cake. But first you have to bake the cake. As you choose exercises from a reference book or discuss possibilities with a trainer, keep this priority in mind. There will be plenty of time to work all the minor muscles in your body—*after* you've established a base level of fitness and conditioned the major groups. These are the groups:

Chest	Back	Shoulders	Arms	Legs	Abdominals

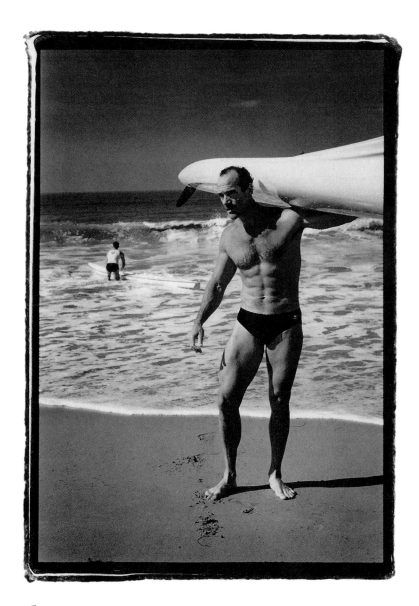

seek symmetry

Mike Newman of *Baywatch* fame has
achieved a near-perfect balance of opposing
muscle groups.

To keep your body in balance and to maintain good posture, avoid joint problems, and minimize injuries, it's always a good idea to exercise *opposing* major muscle groups equally. Like a suspension bridge, the skeleton is held in dynamic tension, but instead of steel cables it is suspended between opposite sets of muscles. If one side is stronger than another, the body's equilibrium is upset, and the whole body feels the effect. If you work the chest muscles, for example, but ignore the upper back, you will end up with round shoulders or sagging posture. If you have an inflexible and strong lower back but weak abdominals, your spine's natural curvature will be altered, and you will likely have a lifetime of back problems. Sometimes the best thing you can do to improve your back is to work on your stomach! Or, if your chest appears recessed and small, you may need to lift and support it by working your middle and upper back. If you think of the analogy of a suspension bridge, it all makes perfect sense.

Here are some major opposing muscle groups:

Chest/Shoulders–Middle/Upper Back
Abdominals–Lower Back
Quadriceps–Hamstrings
Biceps–Triceps

"There is no one routine or combination of exercises that is best for everyone."

If you are new to resistance training, the following eight-week programs will give you an idea of how to get started. For each muscle group in the programs, consult an encyclopedic reference book (Bill Pearl's *Getting Stronger,* for instance) or a knowledgeable person at your local gym. Experiment to see what works best and feels good to you. For every muscle group I have listed below, there are hundreds of exercises. Think of designing your program as an adventure. Your body has its own idiosyncrasies, and part of the fun is in discovering what particular exercises give you the best contraction and the best results. I have resisted prescribing specific exercises for three reasons. First, I want you to understand certain important principles that should inform *any* workout program. Second, I don't want to suggest that there is any single set of exercises that are best—there is no one routine or combination of exercises that is best for everyone. Third, I want you to be responsible for finding your own way down the road to fitness. No one is going to walk the road for you. This book can only get you started.

Resistance Training for Beginners

First 8-Week Program

Muscle	Week 1	Week 2	Week 3	Week 4	Week 5	Weeks 6-8
Abdominals 2 exercises	1 set each 15-20 reps	1 set each 10 reps	2 sets 10 reps	2 sets 10 reps	3 sets 10 reps	3 sets 10 reps
Legs 2 exercises	1 set each 15-25 reps	2 sets each 10 reps	2 sets 10 reps	3 sets 10 reps	3 sets 10 reps	1 set 10 reps
Chest 1 exercise	1 set each 20-30	2 sets each 10 reps	3 sets 10 reps	3 sets 10 reps	1 set 10 reps	1 set 10 reps
Back 1 exercise	1 set each 20-35	3 sets each 10 reps	3 sets 10 reps	1 set 10 reps	1 set 10 reps	2 sets 10 reps
Shoulders 1 exercise	1 set each 25-40	3 sets each 10 reps	1 set 10 reps	1 set 10 reps	2 sets 10 reps	2 sets 10 reps
Triceps 1 exercise	1 set each 30-50	1 set 10 reps	1 set 10 reps	2 sets 10 reps	2 sets 10 reps	3 sets 10 reps
Biceps 1 exercise	1 set each 10 reps	1 set 10 reps	2 sets 10 reps	2 sets 10 reps	3 sets 10 reps	3 sets 10 reps

Notes

- Don't increase weight until third week.
- After third week, increase weight so that last rep is always difficult.
- Train two days per week, with rest day between workouts.
- This workout should take approximately forty-five minutes.
- Do the exercises in order shown (large muscle groups first, followed by small muscle groups).

"Discipline is the natural, almost effortless, result of activities we like to engage in."

For beginners, strength training requires equal parts of discipline and organization. If you want to go for a run, all you have to do is put your jogging shoes on and head out the door. But if you want to do a weight routine, you'll probably have to pack some clothes and go to a gym. For most beginners, going to a gym will require a change in day-to-day life. This is where the discipline comes in. You have to make time in your day, and you have to resist the temptation to fill that time with something else. Remember, fitness is a lifestyle, and you will need to make accommodations in your daily routine from here on out—hopefully, for the rest of your life! One fitness researcher, D. N. Knapp, suggests that making alterations in your lifestyle—establishing new exercise habits—takes about six weeks on average and involves three steps:

- Make the decision to take up weight training
- Make time for the activity
- Maintain a long-term commitment

"A weight-training program, like aerobic work, can be meditative and stress relieving."

Discipline is a word that makes beginners uncomfortable: It seems synonymous with effort and drudgery, not enjoyment or pleasure. If you feel this way about discipline, try thinking of it in a different light. Discipline is the natural, almost effortless, result of activities we like to engage in. If you want to have discipline in your strength-training program, find a routine that you enjoy and *want* to do. If you have pleasure in your workout, it will be self-motivating and self-sustaining. When you first start a strength-training program, it's as important to condition your mind and spirit as your body. Along with learning the correct form of a particular exercise, it's vital to pay attention to what's going on inside, too—how you're feeling and what you're thinking. Search until you find a workout that feels right and is satisfying. If you're doing a routine, and a voice inside says "I hate this," try something different.

A weight-training program, like aerobic work, can be meditative and stress relieving. This is one reason it is important for beginners to ease into their routines. People who pray or meditate regularly learn to quiet their minds first, and then enter into a prayerful or meditative state. Similarly, a warm-up and stretch prepares both the body and the mind for the workout to follow. If you rush into a gym and tear through an exercise routine, you'll miss many of the inner benefits and put yourself at risk for injury, and you'll probably burn out in a few weeks. Strive to make your strength-training program the kind of positive addiction I talked about in chapter 4. Remember, resolve is never enough to keep people going—passion is what counts in the long run;

Resistance Training for Advanced Beginners

Second 8-Week Program

Muscle	Week 1	Week 2	Week 3	Week 4	Week 5	Weeks 6-8
Abdominals 3 exercises	1 set each 15-20 reps	2 sets each 10 reps	3 sets each 10 reps	3 sets each 10 reps	3 sets 10 reps	3 sets 10 reps
Legs 2 exercises	1 set each 15-25 reps	3 sets each 10 reps	3 sets each 10 reps	3 sets each 10 reps	3 sets 10 reps	2 sets 10 reps
Chest 2 exercises	1 set each 20-25	3 sets each 10 reps	3 sets each 10 reps	3 sets each 10 reps	2 sets 10 reps	1 set 10 reps
Back 2 exercises	1 set each 20-25	3 sets each 10 reps	3 sets each 10 reps	2 sets 10 reps	1 set 10 reps	3 sets 10 reps
Shoulders 1 exercise	2 sets each 20-25	3 sets each 10 reps	2 sets each 10 reps	2 sets 10 reps	3 sets 10 reps	3 sets 10 reps
Triceps 1 exercise	2 sets each 20-25	2 sets each 10 reps	2 sets each 10 reps	3 sets 10 reps	3 sets 10 reps	3 sets 10 reps
Biceps 1 exercise	2 sets each 10 reps	2 sets each 10 reps	3 sets each 10 reps	3 sets 10 reps	3 sets 10 reps	3 sets 10 reps

Notes

- Don't increase weight until second week.
- After second week, increase weight so that last rep is always difficult.
- Train three days per week, with rest day between workouts.
- This workout should take approximately sixty minutes.
- Do the exercises in order shown (large muscle groups first, followed by small muscle groups).

and passion comes from the inside. Strength training can be mind-numbing, boring, and repetitious without an inner commitment. Or, it can be a joy, an adrenaline high, and a release from the day's tensions.

A simple way to organize your program and maintain discipline is to keep a workout journal. Write down what you do for each training session, what exercises you like and dislike, how you feel physically and emotionally, and any other information that seems pertinent. Some people like to record their key measurements, like waist and hip size, or (if you're macho) the circumference of their biceps. You could use the same journal to record your aerobic workouts and what you ate that day. Become your own research subject, noting how all the various factors in your life contribute to how you feel on any given day. Your workout journal can become a rich source of information on your journey of fitness. Did you feel strong one day and tired the next? Is there a correlation between what you ate, the aerobic work you did, the amount of sleep you had the night before, or what was going on at the office—or at home? Is your weight up while your measurements are down? Your journal can provide the information you need to answer these questions.

> "Your workout journal can become a rich source of information on your journey of fitness."

A workout card can help you keep track of your daily progress and serve as adjunct to your journal. It can also serve as a reminder of the specific exercises you do from week to week. Here is a simple workout card you can photocopy or use as a guide to design your own.

Personal Workout Card

EXERCISE	Week 1			Week 2			Week 3			Week 4		
	Sets	Reps	Weight	Sets	Reps	Weight	Sets	Reps	Weight	Sets	Reps	Weight
1												
2												
3												
4												
5												
6												
7												
8												
9												
10												
11												
12												

Personal Workout Card

EXERCISE	Week 5			Week 6			Week 7			Week 8		
	Sets	Reps	Weight	Sets	Reps	Weight	Sets	Reps	Weight	Sets	Reps	Weight
1												
2												
3												
4												
5												
6												
7												
8												
9												
10												
11												
12												

Resistance Training
For Intermediate and Advanced Athletes

Once you have established a base level of fitness a whole new world of possibilities opens up. Most people who embrace fitness as a lifestyle are anxious to move onward and upward. There is something deeply empowering about muscular fitness. When you begin to feel your body growing stronger, you seem more capable and powerful in every aspect of your life. I see it all the time with my clients. After a while they begin thinking, "I wonder what I really *can* do?" Two of the things you can do are incorporate more variety in your workouts and experience higher intensity in your routines. You can add sets, repetitions, and weight and utilize more advanced techniques. Here are some elements of intermediate and advanced training you may want to consider for your own workouts.

Supersets.

A superset is two consecutive sets of exercises that work the same muscle or opposing muscles. In a superset, one set of exercises is immediately followed by a second, with no rest in between. After the two exercises are completed, a rest of one or two minutes is taken before resuming the same series. If you are supersetting a single muscle group, the idea is to completely exhaust that muscle and recruit as many muscle fibers as possible. If you are supersetting opposing muscles, the point is to save time while maintaining a near-aerobic heart rate. A variation on the superset is the so-called tri-set or giant set. A superset can include as many continuous sets and exercises as you like.

Pyramids.

A pyramid begins with a low-weight/high-repetition set of exercises, followed by a continuous series of (four to six) sets in which you gradually add weight and decrease repetitions, eventually ending with a high-weight/low-repetition set. A typical pyramid might start out with twelve reps at a light weight and progress to the maximum weight you can lift for a single repetition.

Breakdowns.

The opposite of a pyramid is a breakdown set (sometimes called a multi-poundage set). With a breakdown set, you work your way to the maximum weight you can lift (for six to ten reps) and, after you've exhausted the muscle, remove some of the weight and immediately do another set. When you've completed the lighter set you remove additional weight and do another set, and so on. You can do from one to four sets, "breaking down" the weight each time. Like a pyramid, the point is to completely exhaust the muscle.

Negative Reps.

Weight training loads muscles in two ways. When you contract a muscle and raise a weight, the movement is called a *concentric* motion. When you lower a weight, and your muscle is lengthening rather than contracting, it's called an *eccentric* motion. Negative reps put maximum stress on the eccentric phase of the movement. To do a negative rep, your workout buddy helps you to raise the weight (usually heavy), and you resist the weight, lowering it down as slowly as possible. Your muscles can produce more resistance in the eccentric phase than in concentric, so it's possible to load the muscle with great intensity. This is not for beginners!

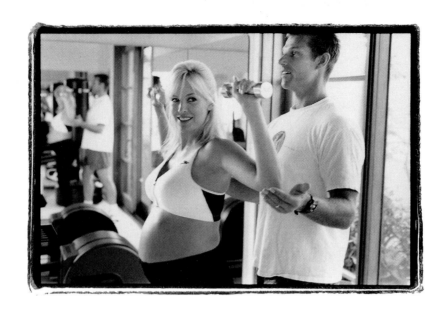

Assisted Reps.

These are also called forced reps and require your workout partner to help you squeeze out a few more repetitions after you've reached the point of exhaustion. The trick here is for your partner to provide just enough assistance so you can complete the full range of motion, but no more. Assisted reps help you to recruit those last few unused muscle fibers.

Split Routines.

Split routines work a particular muscle group (or groups) on one day, and another on the next. A split routine might work the chest and back one day, arms and legs the next, abs the next, and so on. Split routines allow you to work on successive days while still giving your muscles the time they need to rest, recover, and grow.

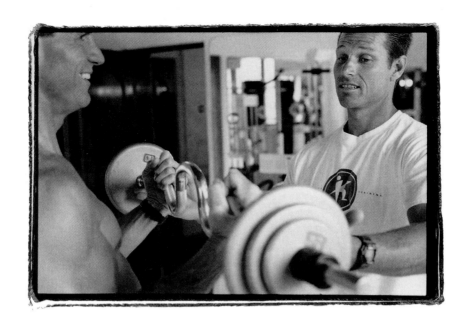

Cycling.

Cycling or cycle training (also called periodization) is an advanced technique in which you train in four periods of four to eight weeks each. Cycle training was first popular in the old Soviet Union and has now been used in the United States for more than a decade. Cycle-training can work for people of all fitness levels, but has been used to greatest effect by athletes in high-strength sports. A typical four-cycle routine of resistance training would look like this:

Cycle 1:	4 to 8 weeks of low weight/high reps
Cycle 2:	4 to 8 weeks of medium weight/medium reps
Cycle 3:	4 to 8 weeks of high weight/low reps
Cycle 4:	4 to 8 weeks of very high weight/low reps or 1 to 2 weeks of active rest (low weight/low reps)

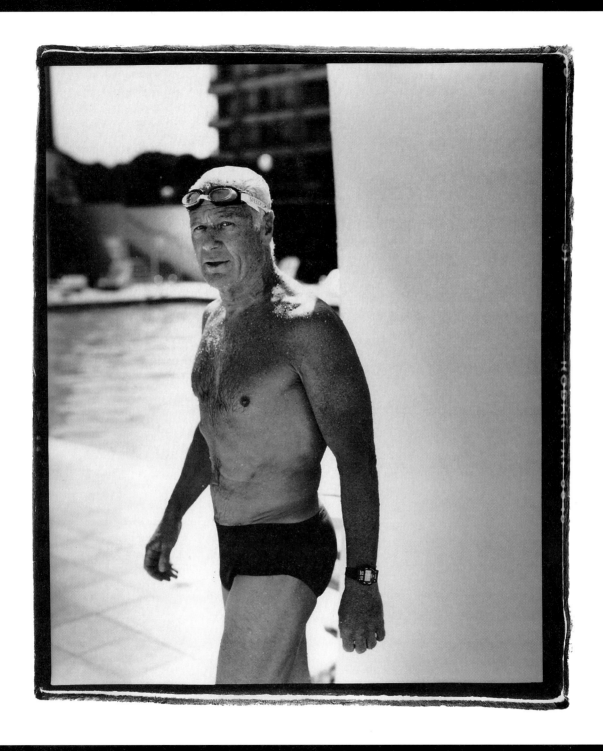

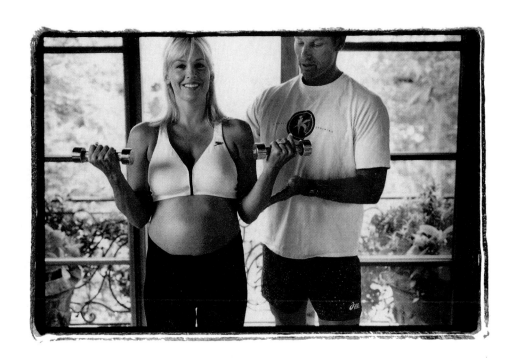

seek pleasure

Discipline is the natural result of an exercise program you enjoy. If you have pleasure in your workout, it will be self-motivating and self-sustaining.

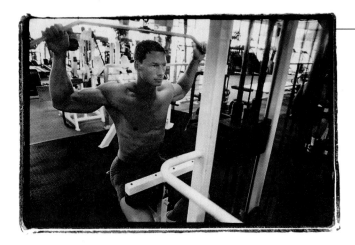

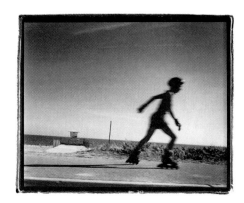

Plyometrics.

Plyometric exercise is popular with athletes who require speed and explosive power. Plyometrics is used in conjunction with regular weight training and often uses body weight or gravity for resistance. A typical exercise would involve jumping from a stationary position back and forth over a hurdle, in a continuous cycle, concentrating on the explosive power necessary to clear it. Or to build chest, arm, and shoulder strength, you might play high-repetition catch with a heavy medicine ball, exploding with each toss. Plyometrics are popular among track and field athletes.

Aerobic Circuit Training.

Aerobic circuit training is an advanced technique that builds endurance and muscle definition. After a good warm-up and stretch, resistance exercises are alternated with aerobic exercises at a very fast pace, with the idea in mind of keeping the heart rate well up into the aerobic zone—right on the edge of anaerobic. For example, if you're working the chest, you would alternate a set of chest exercises with ninety seconds of jumping rope or pedaling at a high RPM on a stationary bike. Everything is done at a high rate of speed. The exercises are done with light weight, twenty to thirty repetitions, as fast as you can. A heart-rate monitor is essential for this kind of workout.

No matter what level of fitness you have achieved, or what type of program you pursue, consistency is the key. But what if you can't always be consistent? What if you go on vacation or get sick? Don't worry. If you are working out, you won't begin to lose any strength for almost six weeks after interrupting your weight-training routine. Some studies have shown that if you work out, you will retain half of your new strength for up to a year after you stop training. When you use muscles regularly, strength declines very slowly, more slowly than with aerobic fitness.

One final reminder about strength training—it's never too early or too late to begin. The earlier you begin, the greater the reserve of muscle mass and bone density you will build for later in life. Those reserves will pay great dividends as you grow older. If you're already a middle-aged baby boomer or senior citizen, don't put it off another day. As unlikely as it may seem, the older you get, the more important strength training becomes. You can gain strength at any age. And that strength will help keep you young.

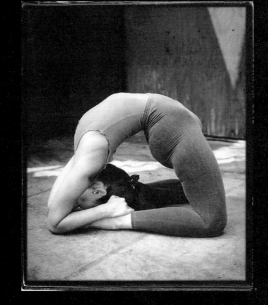

ALTERNATIVES

Madonna has been my number one client for years now. She has turned out to be the perfect practitioner—the ideal disciple—of the philosophy I had been honing over the years with Sean and my other clients. Madonna is not interested in cosmetics, she is interested in fitness and health. She turned out to be the hardest working person I have ever known, and the best "body of work" I could possibly have in my portfolio. Training Madonna was the beginning of an adventure the likes of which I never could have imagined!

CHOOSE YOUR OWN PATH

A sure sign of maturity is an ever increasing awareness of how little we know. In one sense fitness is a young discipline—as a science it hasn't been around very long. But in another sense it is the continuation of a very old pursuit—millennia old. Some of us who promote and teach fitness have come to understand that many of the "new" insights we are learning are not new at all. In fact, in some cases, we are not discovering but *re*-discovering what was already known, practiced, and perfected thousands of years ago. We haven't invented fitness in America, or in this generation. We have much to learn from other cultures, both ancient and modern. And we have something to learn from our own society's heretics, too—those who challenge conventional concepts. Familiarity is often confused with orthodoxy, and orthodoxy

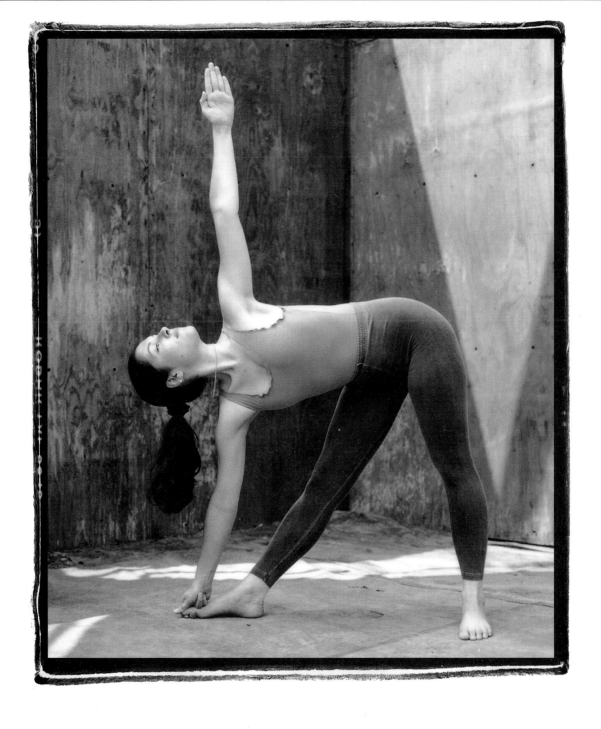

with truth. Yet no single tradition or approach to health has a monopoly on truth. Unfamiliar and unusual approaches to fitness often preserve or advocate important insights.

"No single tradition or approach to health has a monopoly on truth."

Curiosity and an open mind should be our constant companions on the road to fitness. There are many traditions and techniques that seem strange to the Western mind, or too far out of the mainstream to merit our consideration. But it is often the non-Western tradition or the unconventional approach—the ones that challenge our preconceived notions—that hold out the most opportunity for learning and growth. As I have made clear in this book, I hold to the idea that in fitness, as in life, progress depends on becoming a pilgrim, a seeker. In addition to the more conventional paths to fitness, there are many other alternatives, and I encourage my clients to pursue any path that leads them forward on their journey. I'm not advocating an uncritical acceptance of every fitness alternative. Not all approaches are of equal value. Some are merely ludicrous, while others are actually harmful. The legion of "health" books on the market include everything from diets keyed to blood type, to exercise programs based on astrological signs. But don't be put off by the charlatans and health hucksters. Use your good judgment and seek those insights that are rooted in age-old wisdom or new scientific perspectives. All of us need to be responsible stewards of our own health. You must choose your own path.

ALTERNATIVE TRAINING TECHNIQUES

Yoga

One alternative path Madonna has chosen to pursue is Hatha yoga. Hatha yoga and other yogic traditions, challenge us to expand our own culture-bound definition of fitness. It calls into question common American conceptions of fitness by reminding us that true health is not concerned primarily with physical appearance or solely on the body and its physiological processes. Rather, health is about vitality; about growing strong from the inside out. Yoga teaches us that it's a mistake to think of fitness exclusively in terms of muscular strength or aerobic fitness—although both are important. Genuine health is more than going to the gym, or for a run, or having low body fat. True fitness is comprehensive; it is concerned with the mind and the soul, as well as the body. Genuine health, according to the yogic tradition, involves your whole being and involves the balancing of one's inner power or life force with one's physical processes. This idea is the distillation of thousands of years of reflection and practice, and is represented in a variety of

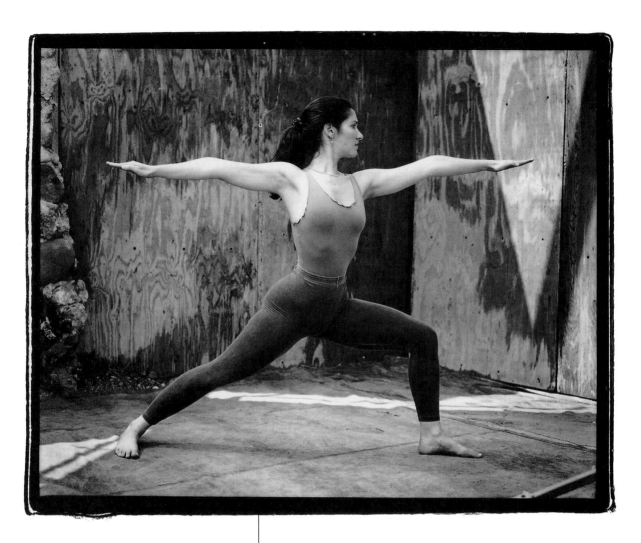

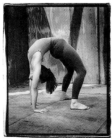

genuine health

Yoga strives to build health from within, at the

deepest level of our being.

ancient cultures. This inner power is called *prana* in India, *chi* in China, *ki* in Japan, and *mana* in Polynesia. The principal goal of Hatha yoga is the development and nurture of a calm and peaceful vitality.

"Yoga reminds us that health has many aspects."

Yoga was developed thousands of years ago. Among the techniques and practices it has developed and refined are many physical routines made up of exercises called *asanas*. These *asanas* were developed to cleanse and detoxify the body, to create and enhance endurance, to facilitate concentration and inner focus, to build strength, and to improve flexibility. Yoga strives to promote growth from within, at the deepest level of our being. Its goal is balance—of the body and psyche. And balance is something desperately needed by many fitness enthusiasts and athletes. For example, tennis players rely on one arm, and basketball players almost always push off from one side. Runners may have strong hearts and lungs, but they may be stiff and inflexible. The price of many otherwise healthy physical pursuits may be an unbalanced body, one unsuited to the performance of common, everyday tasks. An important benefit of yoga is the ability to address these imbalances. Yoga reminds us that health has many aspects, only a small number of which are recognized by most Americans. When we think of yoga we often associate it with a series of postures (the *asanas*). These postures are only one part of yogic practice, but they have significant benefits. The *asanas* and other techniques of yoga are intended to improve physical health and cultivate a calm and peaceful mental state, one that allows for spiritual reflection and self understanding.

"The moment we start connecting to our breath, we connect with life itself."

For many people, yoga can provide the basis on which real strength and fitness is built. We can't perform at our best if we are inflexible, unable to breathe deeply, or uncentered. Health from a yogic perspective is fully integrated. Yoga teaches a form of stretching that is sometimes strenuous, but never stressful. Working from a calm center, stretching should be peaceful and noncompetitive, although it is often rigorous and challenging. Stretching has a contemplative aspect in yoga, in which the practitioner learns to feel and experience the body in direct and unmediated ways. Breath awareness is essential—according to Denise Kaufman, Madonna's yoga teacher—because we can directly influence the flow *prana* (life force) through the flow of our breath. When we learn to cultivate deep, rhythmic breathing, energy blocks in the body are released. As a result, we relieve stress and become more self aware. According to Denise, the value of conscious breathing cannot be underestimated. "The moment we start connecting to our breath, we connect with life itself," she says. Breath is a direct connection to one's mental state and inner being. In yogic teaching, breath control is a means to an end, and that end is to enhance the flow of energy in your body, to reduce physiological imbalances, and to focus your power of attention. This power can then be harnessed in the pursuit of athletic excellence and inner peace.

flexibility

Stretching is sometimes strenuous, but never stressful. Stretching should be peaceful, relaxing, and noncompetitive.

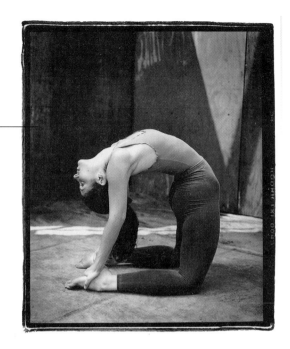

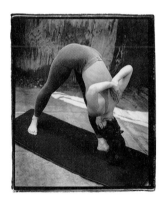

a calm center

Stretching has a contemplative aspect in which we experience our bodies in direct and unmediated ways.

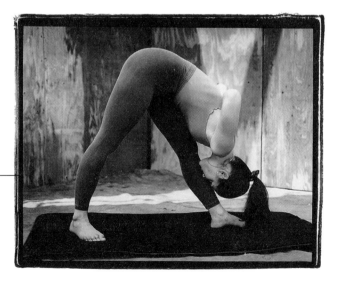

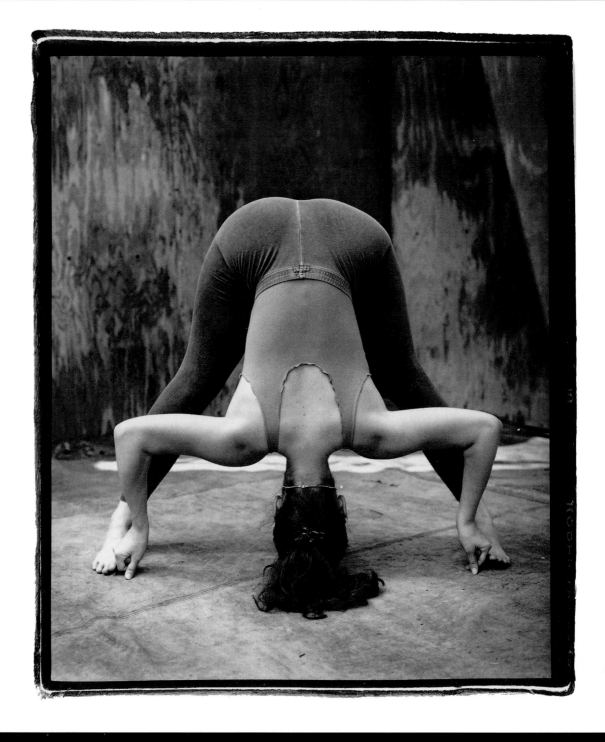

"Yoga develops strength combined with flexibility and balance."

If we are centered, fitness becomes more than the measure of how fast we can run, how much weight we can lift, or how good at a particular sport we can be. This is not to say that yoga is easy. Kareem Abdul Jabar, one of Denise Kaufman's former students, loved to take his buddies to a yoga class and watch them sweat. "They die after the first fifteen minutes!" he used to say with considerable amusement. Yoga can be very strenuous. Madonna's yoga program certainly is. Yoga develops strength combined with flexibility and balance. Madonna's fitness regimen combines the weight training and aerobic work we do together, with yogic strength building, breathing, and flexibility routines. Her high level of fitness and excellent flexibility allow her to pursue a particularly vigorous yogic regimen. But there are many different forms of yoga and as many teachers as there are disciplines. If you choose to explore yoga as a fitness alternative, I encourage you to look at a variety of programs and approaches and see what is best suited to your personal needs and goals. Keep in mind that yoga is not for those who seek quick, dramatic results. The full range of benefits you can experience through yoga practice requires a long-term commitment. However, from your very first session, you should begin to feel both energized and relaxed.

Pilates

In the 1920s Joseph Pilates invented a system of movement and exercise with the goal in mind of strengthening and stretching the muscles, and integrating the mind and body. Pilates, the proverbial skinny, sickly kid, was born in Germany in 1880. His interest in the human body began with his own physique, and by the time he was an adult he had conditioned his body into a strong, lithe, athletic form. He eventually enjoyed success as a gymnast and bodybuilder. During World War I, Pilates was a prisoner of war in England. He passed the war years there inventing spring-driven machines to aid in the reconditioning of wounded soldiers. After the war he continued his work of invention in Germany and eventually moved to New York. Using a variety of ropes, pulleys, and springs, he devised a series of movements and exercises that helped people recover from disease and injury. Over the years, Pilates's original ideas were expanded beyond rehabilitation into a comprehensive fitness program that has been widely used by professional dancers and athletes, but has remained relatively unknown to the general public. During the last decade, however, it has become popular as an alternative form of exercise.

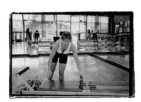
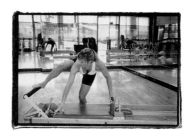
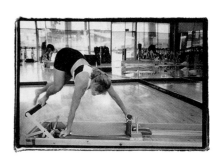

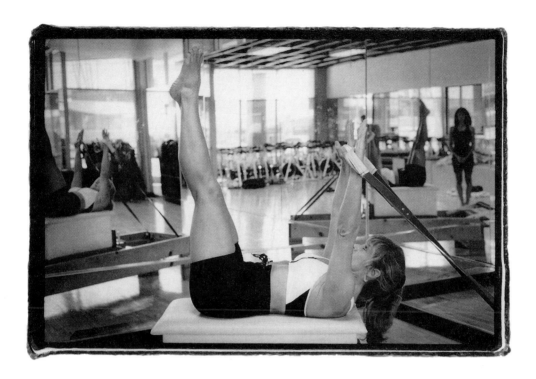

getting centered

Pilates is focused on what dancers and martial artists call the center. The center is located in the pelvic area and is the origin and locus of all movement.

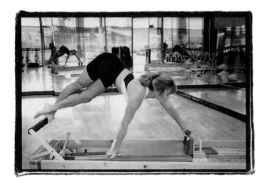

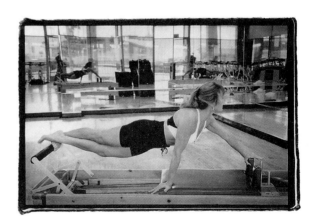

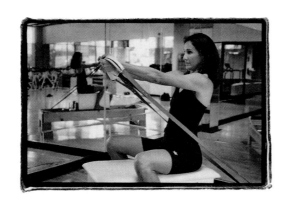

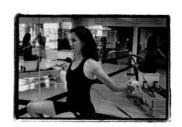

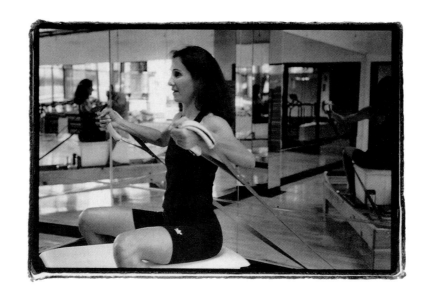

"When we know and experience our center, balance and posture improve, and movement becomes more fluid and economical."

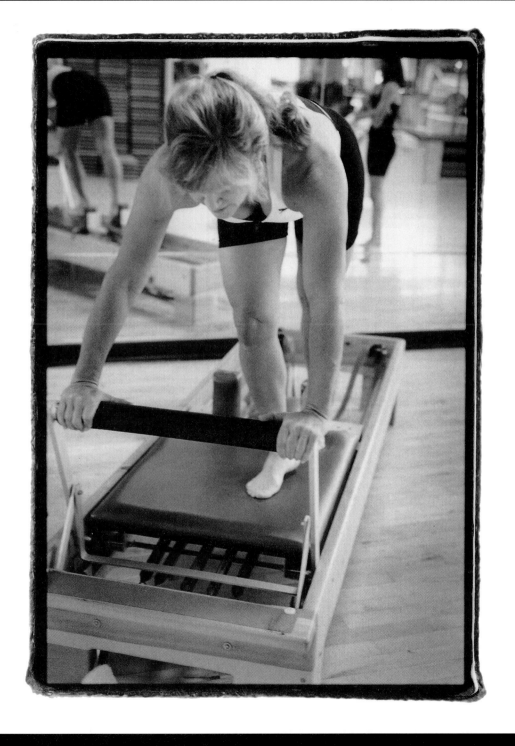

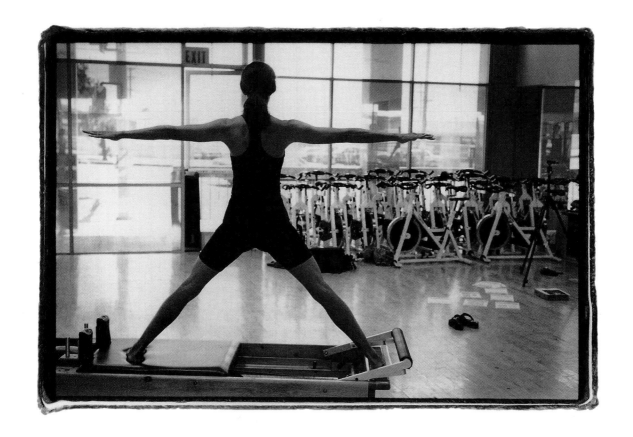

Pilates is similar in some ways to yoga, in that it seeks harmony between the mind and the body. But it is less philosophical and more "Westernized" in its approach. Pilates's exercises seek to work the body from the inside out, beginning with the deep structural muscles of the diaphragm, pelvis, lower back, and buttocks, and then working up and out to the muscles of the chest, shoulders, upper back, and extremities. Pilates is focused on what dancers and martial artists call the "center." The center is located in the pelvic area and is the origin and locus of all movement. When we know and experience our center, balance and posture improve, and movement becomes more fluid and economical.

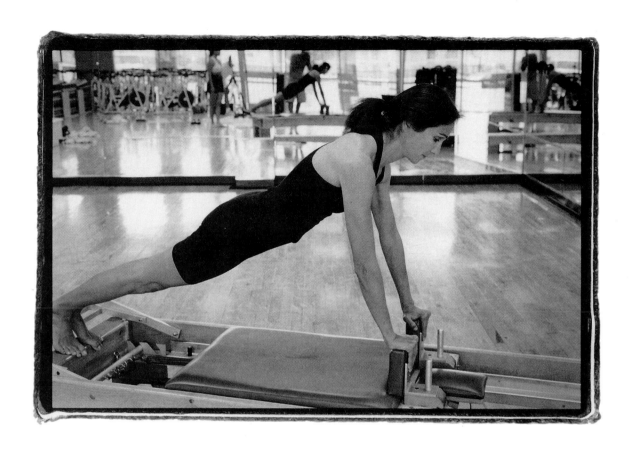

Pilates can be of significant benefit to many typical gym rats who are unbalanced and inflexible, and whose physical stance and gait reflect the fact. Pilates provides a structured way to balance opposing muscle groups, enhance flexibility, and strengthen deep muscles that are otherwise difficult to work.

"One of the benefits of good placement (along with good flexibility) is a dramatic reduction in injuries."

Pilates is usually taught in two contexts. The first is "mat" class, in which the student learns to stretch, exercise, and breathe, while sitting or reclining on a mat on the floor. The only apparatus ordinarily used in a mat class is the mat itself, a thick rubber band, and a small rubber ball. The mat is used for padding, and the rubber band for stretching and resistance movements. The rubber ball is used to teach students how to contract and hold the abdominal muscles. Students learn to draw their abdominal muscles in toward the spine (while on their back) and keep the ball on their stomachs while performing a series of exercises. It's hard at first and can be humiliating! In addition to mat classes, Pilates is also taught on a machine called the "Reformer." The Reformer is an odd-looking device (it looks like a bed designed by the Marquis de Sade) with straps, springs, bungee cords, pulleys, and a sliding seat/platform and is a direct descendant of the hospital contraptions invented by Joseph Pilates. The machine can be used for hundreds of different exercises, many of them deceptively difficult. A good Pilates instructor will use the machine as an aid in assessing a person's strengths and weaknesses, and then as a tool to address those weaknesses.

"Pilates, like yoga, can be used as an adjunct to a fitness program that includes weight training and aerobic exercise, or it can be the main focus of a program. It is not, however, aerobic."

Pilates's techniques have been used with very good results by the San Francisco and New York ballet companies, by many world-famous dancers, and now by an increasing number of professional athletes and actors. Pilates seems to be a particularly effective tool for teaching proper body placement and alignment. One of the benefits of good placement (along with good flexibility) is a dramatic reduction in injuries.

Feldenkrais

Another fitness alternative, and one I have been exploring recently, is based on the work of an Israeli physicist and engineer, Moshe Feldenkrais. Feldenkrais, who died in 1984, was a scientist who became fascinated with the dynamics of human movement. His original motivation was a nagging knee injury. He began to wonder if it was possible to cure his ailing joint by treating it as a biomechanical problem that could be solved by learning (or relearning) to walk correctly. Feldenkrais had a good understanding of body mechanics and joint dynamics from a lifetime of practicing jiujitsu and judo. The unusual combination of a hands-on knowledge of joint manipulation gained from the martial arts, an engineering degree from the University of Paris, and a physics degree from the Sorbonne took Feldenkrais in new and unexpected directions. Obsessed with the desire to understand the intricate relationships that exist between human movement, the skeletal system, neurophysiology, and psychology, he eventually developed a method of assessing and correcting biomechanical imbalances. His own stiff and swollen knees served as his first laboratory. As a scientist he speculated that the way to relieve the stress on his knees was to keep them in alignment, so there would be no "shearing forces" (as only an engineer would put it!) to disturb the joint. This basic theoretical insight was the easy part. The hard part was learning how to change the way he moved and walked.

> "We carry in our bodies the record of old injuries, bad habits, occupational hazards, and emotional stress."

Most of us take movement for granted. We don't think about it much; neither are we conscious of the intricacy involved. Ideally, movements are performed by the action of our major muscle groups while smaller, weaker muscles make minor adjustments and corrections. If everything is working right, we move easily and gracefully through the world. Unfortunately, for most of us, everything isn't working right. We carry in our bodies the record of old injuries, bad habits, occupational hazards, and emotional stress. Worse, we're often not conscious of it. We become accustomed to our dysfunction. We experience the pain, to be sure, but not the source of the pain. The muscles, ligaments, and joints that are the cause of the dysfunction are out of our awareness. Feldenkrais discovered that it is possible to teach people, through a sequence of movements, to become aware of the parts of the self that are out of awareness and not moving. These nonaware, nonmoving parts, he discovered, were often responsible for the stress we feel in joints, ligaments, and muscles. By becoming aware of the complex and subtle action of our bodies, we can often reduce or eliminate pain, inflexibility, and other impairments. And by learning how to reduce stress on our bodies, we can assist the natural healing process.

> "By becoming aware of how we hold our neck, or cinch up our shoulders, or clench our teeth, we empower ourselves to change and eliminate unnecessary strain and tension."

In a nutshell, Feldenkrais discovered that by retraining the body's movements, muscle by muscle, it is possible to live a pain-free existence—with the added benefit of learning to be more elegant and graceful in our movements. He believed that when we present the brain with a choice, it adopts the means of motion that is the most efficient and strains the body the least. The essence of the retraining method developed by Feldenkrais is a technique of physically teaching the body—through the gentle, hands-on manipulation of its muscles and joints (Functional Integration)—a more effective means of moving. Because we learn by experience, presenting our brain with a new choice verbally won't work. By means of simple exercises (Awareness Through Movement), a Feldenkrais practitioner enables the student to become aware of his or her movements by *experiencing* those movements and providing the opportunity to learn alternatives. By becoming aware of how we hold our neck, or cinch up our shoulders, or clench our teeth, we empower ourselves to change and eliminate unnecessary strain and tension. The result is an improvement in posture, breathing, and coordination.

Like yoga, Feldenkrais techniques are concerned with mind-body interactions. Learning to relax, to alter habitual patterns, and increase flexibility, and to develop coordination and a new awareness of the body are among the goals of the Feldenkrais method. The experience of people who have tried it are very similar to those who practice yoga: freer breathing, less discomfort, improved relaxation, and a general sense of physical and mental relief. There are differences, however. Feldenkrais (and Pilates) methods are based more on modern, Western, scientific, cultural assumptions. Unlike yoga, it promises immediate results. This is not to say that the two alternatives are mutually exclusive. They are not. They approach many of the same issues and problems, but from considerably different perspectives. You may be comfortable with yoga, Pilates, Feldenkrais—or none of them! At the least, these perspectives teach us that fitness is multi-dimensional, and involves more than exercise and diet. Fitness involves our whole being. These three fitness alternatives—yoga, Pilates, and Feldenkrais—by no means exhaust the many possibilities open to those on the road to health. They do, however, suggest that an entire lifetime is not enough to explore the fitness landscape. There will always be something new to discover.

Keep The Faith

In the first chapter of this book I wrote that the nature of our daily work and existence is written on our physiques; that the imprint of a sedentary lifestyle can be read in one's posture, gait, and carriage. The wisdom of alternative approaches to health is the constant reminder that our neglected bodies *do* serve as repositories for stress, depression, and illness. Yoga, in particular, helps us make the connection between our physical health and our mental and spiritual well-being. But other disciplines teach us the same lesson. It is a lesson we must learn. We cannot live only in our minds, or only in our bodies. There is a high price to pay for a disintegrated life. An integrated person—body, mind, and spirit—is the goal of fitness. You cannot care for your physical body if you do not nurture your mind and spirit, too. In this book I have relied on religious metaphors to convey many of the ideas and concepts that are central to my philosophy of fitness. If you are a religious person, I hope you will make fitness part of your spiritual regimen. If you are not a religious person, I hope you will acknowledge the connection between your psyche and your body. Either way—whatever your commitment—fitness is the key to a long and satisfying life. Get on the journey to fitness—and keep the faith! ☉